Foot and Ankle Surgery

Guest Editor

THOMAS ZGONIS, DPM, FACFAS

PERIOPERATIVE NURSING CLINICS

www.periopnursing.theclinics.com

Consulting Editor
NANCY GIRARD, PhD, RN, FAAN

March 2011 • Volume 6 • Number 1

SAUNDERS an imprint of ELSEVIER, Inc.

W.B. SAUNDERS COMPANY

A Division of Elsevier Inc.

1600 John F. Kennedy Boulevard ● Suite 1800 ● Philadelphia, Pennsylvania 19103-2899

http://www.periopnursing.theclinics.com

PERIOPERATIVE NURSING CLINICS Volume 6, Number 1

March 2011 ISSN 1556-7931, ISBN-13: 978-1-4557-0487-3

Editor: Katie Hartner
Developmental Editor: Donald Mumford

The ideas and opinions expressed in *Perioperative Nursing Clinics* do not necessarily reflect those of the Publisher. The Publisher does not assume any responsibility for any injury and/or damage to persons or property arising out of or related to any use of the material contained in this periodical. The reader is advised to check the appropriate medical literature and the product information currently provided by the manufacturer of each drug to be administered to verify the dosage, the method and duration of administration, or contraindications. It is the responsibility of the treating physician or other health care professional, relying on independent experience and knowledge of the patient, to determine drug dosages and the best treatment for the patient. Mention of any product in this issue should not be construed as endorsement by the contributors, editors, or the Publisher of the product or manufacturers' claims.

Perioperative Nursing Clinics (ISSN 1556-7931) is published quarterly by Elsevier, 360 Park Avenue South, New York, NY 10010. Months of issue are March, June, September and December. Business and Editorial Offices: 1600 John F. Kennedy Blvd., Suite 1800, Philadelphia, PA 19103-2899. Customer Service Office: 11830 Westline Industrial Drive, St. Louis, MO 63146. Periodicals postage paid at New York, NY and at additional mailing offices. Subscription prices are $124.00 per year (domestic individuals), $213.00 per year (domestic institutions), $61.00.00 per year (domestic students/residents), $161.00 per year (international individuals), $245.00 per year (international institutions), and $65.00 per year (International students/residents). Foreign air speed delivery is included in all *Clinics* subscription prices. All prices are subject to change without notice. **POSTMASTER:** Send change of address to *Perioperative Nursing Clinics*, Customer Service (orders, claims, online, change of address): Elsevier Periodicals Customer Service, 11830 Westline Industrial Drive, St. Louis, MO 63146. Tel: 1-800-654-2452 (U.S. and Canada). Fax: 314-523-5170. E-mail: journals customerservice-usa@elsevier.com (for print support); journalsonlinesupport-usa@elsevier.com (for online support).

Reprints. For copies of 100 or more, of articles in this publication, please contact the Commercial Rights Department, Elsevier Inc., 360 Park Avenue South, New York, NY 10010-1710; Phone: (+1) 212-633-3813; Fax: (+1) 212-462-1935; E-mail: reprints@elsevier.com.

Printed in the United States of America.

Contributors

CONSULTING EDITOR

NANCY GIRARD, PhD, RN, FAAN
Nurse Collaborations, Boerne, Texas; Clinical Associate Professor, Acute Nursing Care Department, University of Texas Health Science Center, San Antonio, Texas

GUEST EDITOR

THOMAS ZGONIS, DPM, FACFAS
Associate Professor, Fellowship Director, and Chief, Division of Podiatric Medicine and Surgery, Department of Orthopaedics, University of Texas Health Science Center at San Antonio, San Antonio, Texas

AUTHORS

CLAIRE M. CAPOBIANCO, DPM
Orthopaedic Associates of Southern Delaware, Lewes, Delaware

ZACHARIA FACAROS, DPM
Fellow, Reconstructive Foot and Ankle Surgery; Clinical Instructor, Division of Podiatric Medicine and Surgery, Department of Orthopaedics, University of Texas Health Science Center at San Antonio, San Antonio, Texas

STEVEN P. KISSEL, DPM
Podiatric Surgical Resident, Division of Podiatric Medicine and Surgery, Department of Orthopaedics, University of Texas Health Science Center at San Antonio, San Antonio, Texas

SHIRMEEN LAKHANI, DPM
Podiatric Surgical Chief Resident, Division of Podiatric Medicine and Surgery, Department of Orthopaedics, University of Texas Health Science Center at San Antonio, San Antonio, Texas

MICHAEL G. PALLADINO, DPM, FACFAS
Assistant Professor and Director of Podiatric Surgical Residency Program, Division of Podiatric Medicine and Surgery, Department of Orthopaedics, University of Texas Health Science Center at San Antonio, San Antonio, Texas

VASILIOS D. POLYZOIS, MD, PhD
Chief of Orthopaedic Traumatology, KAT General Hospital, Athens, Greece

CRYSTAL L. RAMANUJAM, DPM
Fellow, Postgraduate Research and Clinical Instructor, Division of Podiatric Medicine and Surgery, Department of Orthopaedics, University of Texas Health Science Center at San Antonio, San Antonio, Texas

JOHN J. STAPLETON, DPM, FACFAS
Associate, Foot and Ankle Surgery, VSAS Orthopaedics, Allentown; Clinical Assistant Professor of Surgery, Penn State College of Medicine, Hershey, Pennsylvania

JUSTIN WADE, DPM
Podiatric Surgical Resident, Division of Podiatric Medicine and Surgery, Department of Orthopaedics, University of Texas Health Science Center at San Antonio, San Antonio, Texas

THOMAS ZGONIS, DPM, FACFAS
Associate Professor, Fellowship Director, and Chief, Division of Podiatric Medicine and Surgery, Department of Orthopaedics, University of Texas Health Science Center at San Antonio, San Antonio, Texas

Contents

mostly the anatomy is undetected or underestimated until late in the acute care setting. Once the anatomy is correctly identified, surgical treatment is usually required for anatomic restoration, with certain cases being emergent on presentation. Preoperative stabilization, operating room setup, and postoperative care are the essential components for a successful outcome.

Postoperative surgical complications have the potential to develop after any procedure, and patients need to weigh the surgical benefits against the possible risks. These risks are usually small, but complications may result from a multitude of reasons, such as systemic illness, adverse reaction to anesthetic drugs, or improper procedure selection. If multiple preexisting conditions exist, collaboration is required between the medical and surgical disciplines for maximal treatment success.

THE CLINICS ARE NOW AVAILABLE ONLINE!

Access your subscription at:
www.theclinics.com

Preface

Foot and Ankle Surgery

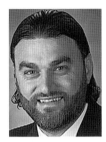

Thomas Zgonis, DPM
Guest Editor

I am honored and grateful to serve as a guest editor for this issue in *Perioperative Nursing Clinics* dedicated to foot and ankle surgery. The purpose of this series is to discuss a broad range of common foot and ankle procedures that are being performed throughout the world. Recent developments and advances within this surgical field have become more globalized among surgeons and health care providers. What is universally understood is that a multidisciplinary team that is well organized and communicates efficiently will provide the best and safest perioperative care to the patient while simultaneously minimizing any potential complications. For these reasons, this unique issue focuses on various topics to better familiarize all health care members of their important role in the patient's successful surgical recovery.

I am also thankful to coauthor and to have most of my current and past surgical residents and fellows from the University of Texas Health Science Center at San Antonio, Texas contribute in this perioperative issue dedicated to all aspects of foot and ankle surgery. The invited authors have provided objective reviews with the highest level of evidence-based practice on the following topics: foot infections, ischemia, Charcot foot reconstruction, orthobiologics, external fixation, rheumatoid arthritis, elective surgery, trauma, soft tissue coverage, and postoperative complications.

A comprehensive approach to the overall well-being of the surgical patient with a strong emphasis on the input of perioperating nursing and health care teamwork is essential for a successful outcome and uneventful patient recovery. Finally, I want to

Perioperative Nursing Clinics 6 (2011) ix–x
doi:10.1016/j.cpen.2010.10.012   **periopnursing.theclinics.com**

thank all the authors for their contributions. I hope that you find this issue beneficial to your daily practice.

Thomas Zgonis, DPM
Division of Podiatric Medicine and Surgery
Department of Orthopaedics
University of Texas Health Science Center at San Antonio
7703 Floyd Curl Drive
Mail Code 7776
San Antonio, TX 78229, USA

E-mail address:
zgonis@uthscsa.edu

Elective Foot and Ankle Surgery

Crystal L. Ramanujam, DPM*, Justin Wade, DPM,
Michael Palladino, DPM

KEYWORDS
- Elective surgery • Foot • Ankle • Perioperative nursing
- Physical therapy

Elective surgical techniques for the foot and ankle are constantly evolving as a result of technological advancement and evidence-based medicine. Proper management by members of the surgical and perioperative nursing teams is based on fundamental principles regarding a thorough knowledge of the patient's medical history, possible complications of the selected surgery, and postoperative rehabilitation.

PREOPERATIVE CONSIDERATIONS

If a period of conservative treatment has failed to alleviate the patient's foot and/or ankle symptoms, elective surgery may be a good option. The patient's chief complaint, physical examination findings, and diagnostic testing must be correlated to enable selection of the best procedure. Detailed discussions between the surgeon and patient regarding the procedures as related to the potential benefits, risks, complications, and postoperative course is imperative. Reasonable expectations for the outcome should be agreed upon far in advance of the surgery. For patients with other medical conditions, clearance from their primary care physician and/or specialists must be obtained to verify that the patient can safely undergo the anesthesia and procedures selected. Diabetic patients must be managed preoperatively with regard to their medications to prevent serious hyperglycemic or hypoglycemic events.[1,2] In patients with rheumatoid arthritis, long-term steroids or immunosuppressive agents should be appropriately tapered to minimize the chance of delayed wound or bone healing.[3] Medications that cause an increased risk of bleeding should be discontinued perioperatively based on procedural selection and recommendations by the patient's primary care physician. Preoperative laboratory testing including complete blood cell count, chemistry profile, coagulation studies, urinalysis, pregnancy test (if indicated), along with chest radiograph and electrocardiogram is the standard procedure in most cases. If abnormal results are found,

Division of Podiatric Medicine and Surgery, Department of Orthopaedics, University of Texas Health Science Center at San Antonio, 7703 Floyd Curl Drive-MSC 7776, San Antonio, TX 78229, USA
* Corresponding author.
E-mail address: Ramanujam@uthscsa.edu

Perioperative Nursing Clinics 6 (2011) 1–7
doi:10.1016/j.cpen.2010.10.004
1556-7931/11/$ – see front matter © 2011 Elsevier Inc. All rights reserved.

appropriate referral for further workup should be made and the elective surgery postponed.

Efforts should be undertaken before surgery to modify risk factors in order to minimize complications. Anesthesia techniques may be modified based on the procedure and the patient's medical history. For example, a patient with a history of rheumatoid arthritis having procedures of short duration, such as hammer toe correction, may have intravenous sedation and local administration of anesthetic rather than risking general endotracheal intubation in a potentially difficult airway. Patients with risk factors for impaired lower extremity circulation should undergo noninvasive vascular laboratory testing. Severe peripheral vascular disease that cannot be improved with revascularization procedures is an absolute contraindication to elective foot or ankle surgery. Knowledge of all revascularization procedures is required for surgical planning, particularly for tourniquet use, incisional approaches, and fixation options. Acute infection at the lower extremity must be addressed before elective procedures. For patients who have preoperative laboratory test results consistent with urinary tract infection, surgery may be delayed to prevent contamination. Smoking cessation in the perioperative period must be encouraged and can be facilitated by formal counseling.[4] Elective procedures may not be undertaken in patients who are nonambulatory, are undergoing active chemotherapy, or have had an acute myocardial infarction in the last 6 months.

Once definitive surgical procedures have been chosen, the surgeon must decide on the equipment required for the procedure, such as instrumentation, hardware, intraoperative fluoroscopy, orthobiologics, hemostasis, suture material, and surgical dressings. Backup or alternative surgical plans should also be in place in case complications are encountered. Direct communication between the surgeon and the scrub technician assigned to the procedures regarding this information is recommended to anticipate all needs. Plans for discharge to home or admission to the hospital after surgery should be discussed in detail with the patient's family or friends. Training for anticipated non–weight bearing with assistive devices by a physical therapist is recommended before the day of surgery.

OPERATIVE SETTING

In the preoperative holding unit, the surgical, anesthesia, and nursing teams must identify and evaluate the patient. Family or other supportive individuals accompanying the patient are identified for contact after the surgery to correctly transport and care for the patient. Verification of the patient's medical/surgical history, allergies, medications taken, and last meal or drink is performed and recorded. A thorough review of the corrective operative limb with marking and all procedures based on the documented informed consent are done by both the surgeon and circulating nurse. The anesthesiologist may begin sedation intravenously with local or regional nerve blocks in the preoperative holding area. The nursing staff helps expedite proper setup of the operating room in advance for the optimal placement of the operating table, anesthesia equipment, and back table with instrumentation and for the provision of adequate room to accommodate intraoperative fluoroscopy and/or arthroscopy equipment to be used when indicated. The patient is transported to the operating room where the nursing staff assist in safe transfer of the patient onto the operating table with proper positioning and securing for the duration of the surgery. In cases of general or spinal anesthesia, intubation or spinal injection, respectively, are performed directly in the operating room. Preoperative weight-based intravenous antibiotics are generally recommended for elective foot and ankle procedures before incision.[5,6] The circulating nurse verbally indicates the name of the patient, operative limb, and procedures, with confirmation from the anesthesia and surgical teams. For surgeries of a longer duration, usually longer than 1.5 hours, segmental compression devices may be placed on the contralateral lower extremity to reduce the risk of venous thromboembolism.[7] A Foley catheter may also be required for long surgical times. A pneumatic ankle, calf, or thigh tourniquet is applied to the operative lower extremity based on the type of anesthesia and the pressure setting based on the patient's blood pressure. Sterile preparation of the operative limb is performed by the circulating nurse with or without assistants, typically using povidone-, iodine-, or chlorhexidine-based solutions and gels; preparation to an area much proximal to the surgical site is required to eliminate contamination.[8] Sterile draping is performed by the surgeon and scrub technician, with frequent observation by the circulating nurse to ensure that sterile precautions are not overlooked. The nursing staff in the operating room should take note of all individuals in the operating room and eliminate unnecessary entry and exit through the operating room doors for the duration of the surgery to reduce contamination of the operative environment.

Because a plethora of elective foot and ankle procedures exist and detailed descriptions for each is beyond the scope of this article, the authors present the following representative procedures with case presentations describing common intraoperative protocols.

Hallux Abducto Valgus Correction

Surgical correction of the hallux abducto valgus (also known as bunion) deformity is one of the most common elective foot procedures performed yet several techniques exist for the variety of types of this abnormality. These procedures are typically divided into groups based on the anatomic location: metatarsal head, metatarsal shaft, or metatarsal base/first metatarsal-cuneiform joint.[9] Oscillating or sagittal saws are usually used for first metatarsal osteotomies and/or ostectomies; however, osteotomes and mallets can be used in lieu of saws. Osteotomy guides have been developed to facilitate accuracy of bone cuts but are used based on surgeon preference. Small fragment screw sets, cannulated or noncannulated, are most commonly used for fixation; however, Kirschner wires, Steinmann pins, or plates (locking or nonlocking) can also be used. Most head and shaft osteotomies can be performed under intravenous sedation with local anesthetic Mayo block. In these cases, ankle or calf tourniquets inflated at 250 or 275 mm Hg, respectively, are used for intraoperative hemostasis after elevation and exsanguination of the surgical lower extremity. More proximal procedures for hallux abducto valgus should be executed under general or spinal anesthesia with the use of a thigh tourniquet typically set at 325 to 350 mm Hg. For arthrodesis procedures at the first metatarsophalangeal joint or first cuneiform joint (Lapidus procedure), large curettes, osteotomes, and allogenic bone grafting material should be available. These arthrodesis procedures are also performed with fluoroscopic guidance; therefore radiology technicians should be informed of their need before the start of the procedure for proper setup. Dressings for most hallux abducto valgus procedures include nonadherent gauze placed directly over the incision site, followed by the application of gauze fluffs and an elastic bandage (**Fig. 1**).

Pediatric Flatfoot Correction

Symptomatic flexible or semiflexible flatfoot can be surgically addressed in children if conservative therapy fails. Procedures in the pediatric population are often performed under general anesthesia and with pneumatic thigh tourniquet. Gastrocnemius recession or Achilles tendon lengthening may be performed to address equinus contracture, which is often a component of these deformities; these techniques are often performed in conjunction with other foot procedures. The patient is brought into the

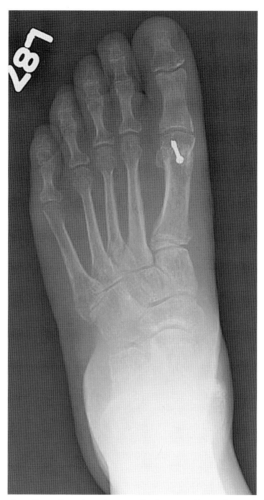

Fig. 1. Anteroposterior view showing the surgical correction of a painful hallux abducto valgus deformity via distal head osteotomy and internal fixation.

operating room and kept on the stretcher where general anesthesia is administered. The operating table is prepared by placing padding for the upper and lower body. The anesthesia, nursing, and surgical teams then carefully flip the patient onto the operating table in the prone position, if needed, taking care of the positions of the head, neck, and arms. Once the tendon lengthening procedure is over, the surgical site is temporarily dressed to protect the area during transition back to the supine position. During these transfer maneuvers, the surgical and nursing staff should constantly be aware of the placement of all intravenous lines, tubing, or other wiring to prevent complications. Symptomatic tarsal coalitions, if present, can be surgically resected, which requires the use of large osteotomes and/or sagittal saw and fluoroscopic guidance. Protection of the patient with a lead shield is a must for pediatric patients. Subtalar joint arthroereisis devices have been developed for the correction of flexible flatfoot deformity, with insertion and removal sets specific to the implant selected.[10] Flatfoot associated with an accessory navicular may require excision and advancement of the posterior tibial tendon (Kidner procedure); for this procedure, plication of the tendon can be done with slowly absorbable suture or with reinforcement using a bone anchor. Rearfoot arthrodesis procedures can be performed, if indicated, in severe cases and often require the use of large curettes, self-retaining retractors, osteotomes, and supplemental allogenic bone grafting. Fixation options include cannulated small and large fragment screw sets and locking or nonlocking plates. Sterile gauze dressings followed by well-padded posterior splints are usually applied at the end of these procedures (**Fig. 2**).

Rearfoot Arthrodesis

Selective arthrodesis of hindfoot joints is indicated for posttraumatic arthrosis, rheumatoid arthritis, or primary arthrosis that is unresponsive to conservative measures.[11] These procedures are performed under general or spinal anesthesia with the patient in supine position and with a pneumatic thigh tourniquet for hemostasis. Foley catheters are often warranted because of lengthy surgical times associated with extensive arthrodesis techniques, particularly when external fixation is used. As described previously, large fragment screw sets, Steinmann pins, plates, washers, external fixation, and bone graft should be available.[12] Careful positioning, use of segmental compression devices to the contralateral lower extremity, and judicious atraumatic technique are essential to minimize complications. Sutures are often reinforced with skin staples for these procedures requiring more extensive incisions. Some surgeons advocate the use of surgical drains in hindfoot arthrodesis; therefore, if chosen, proper precautions should be taken to monitor drainage and remove the device in a timely manner. Sterile gauze dressings and well-padded posterior splints or short leg casts are often used for immobilization after these surgeries. If external fixation is used, appropriate pin site dressings and care are imperative (**Fig. 3**).[13]

POSTOPERATIVE RECOVERY

Postoperative pain control is based on the extent of surgical procedures and patient's level of tolerance. For smaller procedures such as distal first metatarsal osteotomies for hallux abducto valgus correction, administration of oral medication such as hydrocodone for the first 2 postoperative weeks may suffice. If a patient is kept overnight or longer in the hospital for observation, sliding scale intravenous and/or oral pain medication can be used. For extensive procedures involving the rearfoot, ankle, and external fixation, patient-controlled analgesic pumps are helpful to maintain patient comfort for immediate postoperative days. Recovery room or inpatient nurses should monitor the patient's pain levels using the visual analog scale frequently so that treatment can be rendered accordingly. Special attention to total pain medication usage in correlation with symptoms is important. Signs of desaturation secondary to narcotic

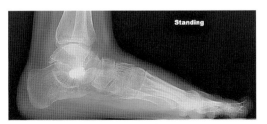

Fig. 2. Lateral view showing the placement of a subtalar joint arthroereisis device for the surgical correction of a pediatric flexible flatfoot deformity.

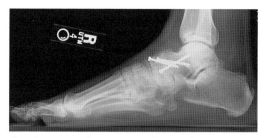

Fig. 3. Lateral view showing surgical correction of a painful posttraumatic arthrosis via isolated talonavicular joint arthrodesis using internal fixation.

overdose should alert nurses for the administration of reversal agents and supportive measures. Nursing staff may also be aware of high levels of pain that do not seem to coincide with that expected from the specific surgical procedure. In these cases, the surgeon should immediately be contacted to examine the patient for possible causes, such as compartment syndrome at the surgical site. Precautions for infection and deep vein thrombosis should entail administration of prophylactic antibiotics and anticoagulants, respectively. First-generation cephalosporins are usually adequate for coverage of organisms most responsible for infections after foot and ankle elective surgery. Nursing staff may also avoid exposure of the surgical sites to prevent contamination and subsequent infection. Subcutaneous daily injection of enoxaparin, use of segmental compression devices, and performing frequent knee flexion exercises are recommended after procedures, which require periods of prolonged immobilization, especially external fixation.

PHYSICAL THERAPY AND REHABILITATION

Progressive physical therapy can be ordered based on the type of foot or ankle surgery performed, anticipated healing time, and individual functional goals. The standard prescription for physical therapy must take into account the ideal time to start the therapy, the patient's ability to safely perform certain modalities, and a specific description of functional limitations, if present. Perioperative nursing staff play a significant role in rehabilitation because their careful observations of the patient can provide clues regarding the patient's capacity to participate in formal physical therapy and also whether therapy is proving effective. The goals of rehabilitation include increased strength and range of motion as well as decreased pain and swelling.[14] A variety of modalities exist at the disposal of the surgeon, which include cryotherapy, thermotherapy, contrast baths, massage, ultrasound therapy, phonophoresis, electrotherapy, and passive and active range of motion exercises.[15] The patient can perform these therapies under the guidance of a physical therapist and will often achieve better overall satisfaction after the elective foot and ankle surgery. Physical therapy may also be useful in the management of chronic regional pain syndrome, if it occurs after a foot and ankle procedure.[16]

SUMMARY

Optimal outcomes for surgical correction of symptomatic foot and ankle conditions are best achieved with a multidisciplinary team approach. Perioperative care of the patient undergoing elective foot and ankle surgery should be tailored according to the procedure, medical status of the patient, and level of progression throughout the course of rehabilitation.

REFERENCES

1. Skully R, Beasley CA, Lutz KW. Current trends in preoperative patient evaluation and management for podiatric surgeons. Clin Podiatr Med Surg 2003;20:213–35.
2. Mehta SK, Breitbart EA, Berberian WS, et al. Bone and wound healing in the diabetic patient. Foot Ankle Clin 2010;15:411–37.
3. Bibbo C, Goldberg JW. Infectious and healing complications after elective orthopaedic foot and ankle surgery during tumor necrosis factor-alpha inhibition therapy. Foot Ankle Int 2004;25:331–5.
4. Krannitz KW, Fong HW, Fallat LM, et al. The effect of cigarette smoking on radiographic bone healing after elective foot surgery. J Foot Ankle Surg 2009; 48:525–7.
5. Okun S, Mehl S, DellaCorte M, et al. The use of prophylactic antibiotics in clean podiatric surgery. J Foot Surg 1984;23:402–6.
6. Zgonis T, Jolly GP, Garbalosa JC. The efficacy of prophylactic intravenous antibiotics in elective foot and ankle surgery. J Foot Ankle Surg 2004;43:97–103.
7. Myerson MS, Henderson MR. Clinical applications of a pneumatic intermittent impulse compression device after trauma and major surgery to the foot and ankle. Foot Ankle 1993;14:198–203.
8. Brooks RA, Hollinghurst D, Ribbans WJ, et al. Bacterial recolonization during foot surgery: a prospective randomized study of toe preparation techniques. Foot Ankle Int 2001;22:347–50.
9. Bai LB, Lee KB, Seo CY, et al. Distal chevron osteotomy with distal soft tissue procedure for moderate to severe hallux valgus deformity. Foot Ankle Int 2010; 31:683–8.
10. Fernández de Retana P, Alvarez F, Viladot R. Subtalar arthroereisis in pediatric flatfoot reconstruction. Foot Ankle Clin 2010;15:323–35.
11. Weinraub GM, Schuberth JM, Lee M, et al. Isolated medial incisional approach to subtalar and talonavicular arthrodesis. J Foot Ankle Surg 2010;49:326–30.
12. Kanakaris NK, Mallina R, Calori GM, et al. Use of bone morphogenetic proteins in arthrodesis: clinical results. Injury 2009;40(Suppl 3):S62–6.
13. Zgonis T, Jolly GP, Blume P. External fixation use in arthrodesis of the foot and ankle. Clin Podiatr Med Surg 2004;21:1–15.
14. Schuh R, Hofstaetter SG, Adams SB Jr, et al. Rehabilitation after hallux valgus surgery: importance of physical therapy to restore weight bearing of the first ray during the stance phase. Phys Ther 2009;89:934–45.
15. Rath S, Schreuders TA, Stam HJ, et al. Early active motion versus immobilization after tendon transfer for foot drop deformity: a randomized clinical trial. Clin Orthop Relat Res 2010;468:2477–84.
16. Duman I, Dincer U, Taskaynatan MA, et al. Reflex sympathetic dystrophy: a retrospective epidemiological study of 168 patients. Clin Rheumatol 2007;26: 1433–7.

Perioperative Care for Rheumatoid Foot and Ankle Surgery Patients

Crystal L. Ramanujam, DPM[a], Thomas Zgonis, DPM[a,b],*

KEYWORDS

- Arthropathy • Synovitis • Arthrodesis • Foot
- Rheumatoid arthritis

Rheumatoid arthritis (RA) is a systemic autoimmune inflammatory arthropathy that affects approximately 1% to 2% of adults worldwide.[1,2] The disease is often debilitating and leads to progressive joint inflammation and destruction, with subsequent functional impairment. The hands and legs are most commonly involved, with women more frequently affected than men, and the most common age groups affected lie between 40 and 60 years. Juvenile RA is the most common form of childhood arthritis, yet its clinical pattern usually differs from that of adult RA. The exact cause of RA is unknown but research points toward a genetic predisposition with certain infections or environmental factors that might trigger the activation of the immune system in susceptible individuals. Immune cells, called lymphocytes, are activated and cytokines, such as tumor necrosis factor (TNF) and interleukins 1 and 6 are expressed in the inflamed areas leading to articular effusions. Synovial hypertrophy contributes to the formation of synovial pannus, which selectively causes destruction to periarticular structures, cartilage, and bone. RA can affect any joint including the hand, wrist, elbow, shoulders, hip, knee, foot, ankle, and cervical spine. Nearly 100% of patients report foot problems within 10 years of RA onset.[3–5] Sites of involvement often coincide with the duration of the disease, with forefoot involvement occurring much earlier than hindfoot or ankle disease (**Fig. 1**).[6]

[a] Division of Podiatric Medicine and Surgery, Department of Orthopaedics, University of Texas Health Science Center at San Antonio, 7703 Floyd Curl Drive, MSC 7776, San Antonio, TX 78229, USA
[b] Research and Reconstructive Foot and Ankle Fellowships, University of Texas Health Science Center at San Antonio, 7703 Floyd Curl Drive, MSC 7776, San Antonio, TX 78229, USA
* Corresponding author. Division of Podiatric Medicine and Surgery, Department of Orthopaedics, University of Texas Health Science Center at San Antonio, 7703 Floyd Curl Drive, MSC 7776, San Antonio, TX 78229.
E-mail address: Zgonis@uthscsa.edu

Perioperative Nursing Clinics 6 (2011) 9–16
doi:10.1016/j.cpen.2010.10.009
1556-7931/11/$ – see front matter © 2011 Elsevier Inc. All rights reserved.

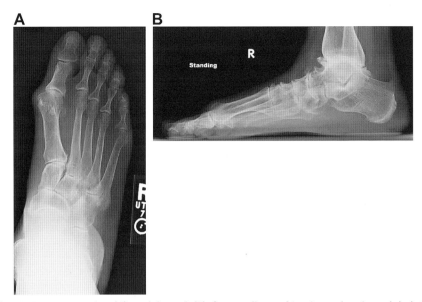

Fig. 1. Anteroposterior (*A*) and lateral (*B*) foot radiographic views showing global RA involvement of the foot and ankle in a female patient. The condition is characterized by periarticular forefoot osteopenia with erosions and edema, hallux valgus deformity, joint space loss, and osteophytosis at the midfoot, hindfoot, and ankle.

INDICATIONS/CONTRAINDICATIONS OF SURGERY

Patients who have chronic painful pedal deformities that are not relieved with conservative measures often seek surgical treatment. Surgical care should be balanced with medical management. The pattern of joint involvement in the foot or ankle and eventual functional goals of the patient must be carefully considered. In general, one must take into account whether the patient is in adequate physical and mental condition to permit surgical intervention. Perioperative collaboration with the patient's rheumatologist and/ or primary care physician is essential to properly manage all aspects of care. In addition, socioeconomic factors should be considered in major reconstructive procedures, especially with regard to the patient's emotional support system for assistance throughout the perioperative period and financial ability to use comprehensive rehabilitation efforts for optimal recovery. Interactive discussions must be undertaken between the patient and surgical team, regarding both the risks and benefits to the selected foot and ankle surgery.

There are a variety of foot and ankle procedures that can be performed to decrease pain, correct deformity, and prevent progression of functional decline. Perioperative care of patients with RA must take into consideration their disease state, medical therapy, and functional status because these factors specifically relate to the selected surgical procedure. Procedures described generally fall under the following categories: joint-sparing methods, resection arthroplasty, implant arthroplasty, or arthrodesis.

Forefoot

The most common forefoot deformity in RA is hallux valgus and lesser digital contractures.[7–11] In early stages of RA, joint-sparing techniques can be performed, such as synovectomy, capsular release, and/or other soft tissue realignment procedures, to delay the progression of joint destruction. By far, the most common procedure reported for forefoot reconstruction is panmetatarsal head resection (**Fig. 2**).[10] It is

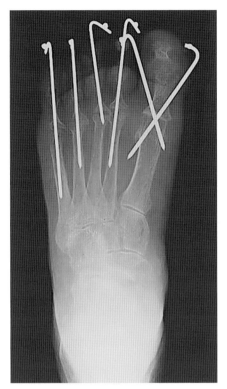

Fig. 2. Anteroposterior radiograph of the foot following panmetatarsophalangeal joint arthrodesis for RA forefoot reconstruction.

recommended that digital deformities be addressed with interphalangeal joint arthrodesis rather than arthroplasty because the latter often leads to recurrence. Resection of the base of the hallux as described by Keller[12] is a popular option for the symptomatic first metatarsophalangeal joint. Metal or silicone implants, total or hemitype, have also been used; however, outcomes have been inconsistent. Complications for these procedures include recurrent deformity, transfer lesions, metatarsalgia, and implant failure.[13,14] Arthrodesis of the first metatarsophalangeal joint for severe arthrosis has the most favorable and predictable outcomes in patients with RA.[15] Arthrodesis of the lesser metatarsophalangeal joints has also been successfully described to correct forefoot abnormality and prevent progression.[16]

Midfoot and Hindfoot

Advanced symptomatic arthrosis of the midfoot, particularly the tarsometatarsal joint complex, is most often treated by selective arthrodesis of the involved joint. Medial column fusion is a good option to correct longitudinal arch deficiency. Rearfoot deformity, most commonly leading to hindfoot valgus, can be addressed through corrective osteotomies, yet fusion is the most reliable option for late-stage arthrosis.[17]

Ankle

Chronic RA can lead to painful symptoms at the ankle, usually secondary to proliferative synovitis and articular damage. Limited arthroscopic debridement or exostectomy can be performed for mild cases. Ankle arthrodesis is best reserved for end-stage debilitating arthrosis. Several methods of correction include internal fixation using screws, plates, staples, pins, and/or intramedullary rods; external fixation; combination of internal and external fixation; and arthrodesis using arthroscopic techniques. Simultaneous arthrodesis can also be performed at the subtalar joint, if clinically indicated. Malunion is the most commonly reported complication of ankle arthrodesis.[18] Total ankle replacement is an option that preserves motion and decreases stress to adjacent joints when compared with ankle arthrodesis. Complications of total ankle replacement for RA include implant failure, infection, fracture, nerve injury, persistent pain, and wound complications. Many patients with RA still require bracing, orthoses, and/or shoe modifications after surgical intervention to provide long-term protection and to prevent complications.

PREOPERATIVE CONSIDERATIONS

A thorough preoperative vascular physical examination in conjunction with noninvasive vascular laboratory testing is recommended for all patients considering foot and ankle surgery for RA. Procedures for deformity correction place patients at risk for vascular compromise because of long-standing contractures, particularly at the forefoot. Patients with RA who may have associated Raynaud phenomenon and/or vasculitis are also more likely to have fragile skin with a predilection for breakdown. Signs of arterial and/or venous insufficiency should be investigated and appropriately addressed before elective foot or ankle surgery. Formal vascular surgical consultation may be warranted in patients with advanced disease, and if any revascularization procedures are performed, coordination of foot or ankle reconstruction should proceed accordingly based on the risk and healing potential. In addition, a history of cardiovascular or cardiopulmonary disease associated with RA may compound surgical risk in terms of how aggressive surgical correction can be and can further affect anesthesia choices and postoperative functional status. Neurologic manifestations seen in RA, typically sensory peripheral neuropathy that is most notable in the lower extremities, may also have a significant impact on surgery selection and outcome because the risk for ulceration and/or infection is higher in these patients.

Depending on the type of foot or ankle surgery, appropriate anesthesia techniques should be considered. Patients with RA who have previously undiagnosed cervical spine disease can have major implications for anesthesia selection if the selection is incorrectly manipulated. Preoperative lateral radiographs of the cervical spine in flexion and extension are a must to evaluate for potential atlantoaxial subluxation. In severe cases, general endotracheal anesthesia may be contraindicated. Similarly, patients with extensive arthrosis of the spine may not be candidates for spinal anesthesia. Several foot and ankle procedures can be performed safely under intravenous anesthesia with local or regional anesthetic blocks.

Most patients with RA take a combination of the following categories of medications: nonsteroidal antiinflammatory drugs (NSAIDs), glucocorticoids, and disease-modifying antirheumatic drugs (DMARDs). All of these drugs may theoretically adversely affect normal inflammatory processes involved in wound and bone healing, therefore potentially affecting surgical outcomes.

With regard to NSAIDs, the decision to stop their use before surgery largely depends on the type and dosage of the medication taken by the patient. The effects of NSAIDs, such as ibuprofen and ketorolac, having reversible effects on platelets are dose dependent; therefore, the decision to continue the medication is based on the type of surgery anticipated, because some procedures may cause more increased risk of bleeding than others. On the other hand, aspirin use should be held at least 5 to

10 days before surgery because of its irreversible effects on platelets and increased risk of bleeding.

Patients on chronic corticosteroid therapy (such as prednisone, prednisolone, and methylprednisolone) should be managed preoperatively based on their usual drug dosage and the level of physiologic stress the surgery may impose.[19] Steroids are the most powerful antiinflammatory agents available today; therefore, their use should be tapered as much as possible. Typically, maintenance of the daily home dose perioperatively is recommended to avoid adrenal insufficiency. On the day of surgery, for most forefoot procedures, 25 mg of hydrocortisone or 5 mg of methylprednisolone should be administered intravenously. For procedures associated with moderate levels of stress, such as rearfoot or ankle reconstructive procedures, 50 to 75 mg of hydrocortisone or 10 to 15 mg of methylprednisolone intravenously is recommended.[20]

The DMARDs encompass a large class of drugs including the following: gold salts, hydroxychloroquine, sulfasalazine, D-penicillamine, and the immunosuppressive agents known as methotrexate (MTX), azathioprine, leflunomide, cyclosporine, and cyclophosphamide. This class differs from NSAIDs and steroids in that they act slowly for a period of 1 to 3 months and they seem to alter the natural history of RA. For patients with moderate to severe disease, MTX has become a central component to therapy because of its ability to control aggressive RA. Continuation of MTX administration throughout the perioperative period is associated with fewer postoperative flares and fewer surgical complications in most patients.[21–23] However, in high-risk patients, cessation of MTX use 1 week preoperation is recommended.[19]

Biologic agents including anti-TNF agents (etanercept [Enbrel]) have become more widespread and are often used in combination with DMARDs. These drugs primarily inhibit the initiation and perpetuation of the proinflammatory molecule TNF-α in rheumatoid synovitis. Overall, anti-TNF agents are associated with an increased risk of infection.[24] Rheumatologists typically recommend ceasing the use of anti-TNF medications at least 2 weeks before surgery.[25]

Preoperative administration of an intravenous weight-based antibiotic directed against staphylococcal and streptococcal bacteria is recommended for all elective rheumatoid foot and ankle procedures because of the increased risk for infection in this population.[19,26]

OPERATIVE SETTING

Appropriate measures should be taken in handling the patient, especially in transferring and positioning throughout the intraoperative period based on the patient's disease status. As previously stated, careful manipulation of the head and neck, as well as padding to bony prominences can prevent complications. Patients who may have severe contractures at the hip or knee should be accommodated accordingly. Decision for lower extremity tourniquet use is based on the type of anesthesia used, type of procedure to be performed, preoperative vascular status of the patient, and length of surgical period. For long procedures, use of a pneumatic compression device for the contralateral limb is recommended to reduce the risk for lower extremity deep vein thrombosis (DVT). The scrub technician and circulating nurse should discuss with surgeons in advance regarding procedures requiring fixation, because multiple options such as screws, pins, plates, and grafting material may be considered and should be available in the operating room in case first-choice techniques cannot be used for reasons such as poor bone quality. Atraumatic techniques should be always performed not only by the surgeon but also by the surgical nursing assistants, facilitating retraction. Avoidance of pressure or tension on the skin at surgical sites is imperative. Pie-crusting techniques can be used to relieve skin tension, and surgical dressings should be light yet protective. Special attention should be given to the patient's heel where adequate soft padding should be applied if using casts or splints.

POSTOPERATIVE CONSIDERATIONS

In the recovery room setting, many precautions are taken to avoid some of the well-known complications of foot and ankle surgery in patients with RA. Postoperative infection rates for these procedures have been reported to range between 5% and 35%.[19,26] Postoperative antibiotics directed against gram-positive bacteria should be continued for cases involving extensive elective reconstruction for 24 to 32 hours duration. For surgeries that have addressed infectious processes, culture-specific intravenous antibiotics are recommended and may require long-term suppressive therapy. Pain control immediately following the surgery can be difficult and requires adjustment based on the procedure and patient's tolerance. Frequent checks by the nursing team are usually required to ensure that analgesics are providing adequate levels of comfort. In cases of rearfoot or ankle reconstruction with internal and/or external fixation, patient-controlled analgesic pumps may be indicated; however, the presence of severe hand deformities may preclude their use. Patients requiring postoperative immobilization or bed rest should be observed carefully to prevent skin pressure lesions.

Postoperative admission to the hospital for observation, pain control, and rehabilitation may be required for certain procedures. Off-loading boots for protection of the heels should be used as needed. Furthermore, frequent turning and changes in position can also prevent DVT. Surgical dressings in patients who have undergone elective procedures should avoid tension against the skin. Nursing personnel may avoid unnecessary dressing changes postoperatively unless directed otherwise by the surgeon; thus, the risk of contamination and infection can be decreased.

Drug therapy for the postoperative period should be based on recommendations from the patient's rheumatologist and/or primary care physician and also must be individualized based on the type of procedure undertaken. NSAIDs have been shown to inhibit bone healing, therefore they should be avoided in the immediate postoperative period following osteotomies or arthrodesis procedures of the foot and ankle. Although use of corticosteroids has also been associated with adverse effects on wound and bone healing, their use must be judiciously balanced in relation to their need to control the patient's systemic RA. Based on risks involved in the immobilization of the lower extremity, DVT prophylaxis is recommended after the first postoperative day and for a period of 2 to 3 weeks following hospital discharge.[8,27]

Rehabilitation of patients with RA is as important as the actual foot or ankle surgical procedures. Quality-of-life considerations in the RA population should focus on therapeutic patient education and physical therapy.[28] Appropriate selection of assistive devices, if needed during non–weight-bearing, is important because limitations can be imposed by rheumatoid involvement of the upper extremities.[29] Newer developments in platform crutches and rolling walkers can allow patients with RA to maintain some mobility, which is important for improvement of both emotional and functional well-being.[30]

SUMMARY

The foot and ankle are involved nearly in all patients with RA. For the medical and surgical personnel participating in the care of such patients who undergo foot or ankle surgery, knowledge of this complex systemic disease process and proper perioperative management are essential for positive outcomes.

REFERENCES

1. Wilder RL. Rheumatoid arthritis: epidemiology, pathology and pathogenesis. In: Schumacher HR, Klippel JH, Koopman WJ, editors. Primer on the rheumatic diseases. 10th edition. Atlanta (GA): The Arthritis Foundation; 1993. p. 86–9.
2. Lorenzo M. Rheumatoid arthritis. Foot Ankle Clin 2007;12:525–7.
3. Jaakkola JI, Mann RA. A review of rheumatoid arthritis affecting the foot and ankle. Foot Ankle Int 2004;25:866–74.
4. Shi K, Tomita T, Hayashida K, et al. Foot deformities in rheumatoid arthritis and relevance of disease severity. J Rheumatol 2000;27:84–9.
5. Loredo R. Radiographic manifestations of rheumatic diseases affecting the foot and ankle. Clin Podiatr Med Surg 1999;16:215–58.
6. Fleming A, Crown JM, Corbett M. Early rheumatoid disease. I Onset. Ann Rheum Dis 1976;35:357–60.
7. Vainio K. The rheumatoid foot: a clinical study with pathologic and rheumatologic comments. Ann Chir Gynaecol 1956;45(Suppl 1):1–107.
8. Vidigal E, Jacoby RK, Dixon AS, et al. The foot in chronic rheumatoid arthritis. Ann Rheum Dis 1975;34:292–7.
9. Grondal L, Tengstrand B, Nordmark B, et al. The foot: still the most important reason for walking incapacity in rheumatoid arthritis: distribution of symptomatic joints in 1,000 RA patients. Acta Orthop 2008;79:257–61.
10. Hoffmann P. An operation for severe grades of contracted or claw toes. Am J Orthop Surg 1912;9:441–9.
11. Raunio P, Laine H. Synovectomy of the metatarsophalangeal joints in rheumatoid arthritis. Acta Rheumatol Scand 1970;16:12–7.
12. Keller WL. The surgical treatment of bunions and hallux valgus. N Y Med J 1904; 80:741–2.
13. Moeckel B, Sculco T, Alexiades M. The double-stemmed silicone-rubber implant for rheumatoid arthritis of the first metatarsophalangeal joint. J Bone Joint Surg Am 1992;74:564–70.
14. Townley C, Taranow W. A metallic hemiarthroplasty resurfacing prosthesis for the hallux metatarsophalangeal joint. Foot Ankle Int 1994;15:575–80.
15. Mann RA, Thompson FM. Arthrodesis of the first metatarsophalangeal for hallux valgus in rheumatoid arthritis. J Bone Joint Surg Am 1984;64:687–92.
16. Jeffries LC, Rodriguez RH, Stapleton JJ, et al. Pan-metatarsophalangeal joint arthrodesis for the severe rheumatoid forefoot deformity. Clin Podiatr Med Surg 2009;26:149–57.
17. Knupp M, Skoog A, Tornkvist H, et al. Triple arthrodesis in rheumatoid arthritis. Foot Ankle Int 2008;29:293–7.
18. Maenpaa H, Lehto MU, Belt EA. Why do ankle arthrodeses fail in patients with rheumatic disease? Foot Ankle Int 2001;22:403–8.
19. Howe CR, Gardner GC, Kadel NJ. Perioperative medication management for the patient with rheumatoid arthritis. J Am Acad Orthop Surg 2006;14:544–51.
20. Lamberts SW, Bruining HA, de Jong FH. Corticosteroid therapy in severe illness. N Engl J Med 1997;337:1285–92.
21. Grennan DM, Gray J, Loudon J, et al. Methotrexate and early postoperative complications in patients with rheumatoid arthritis undergoing elective orthopaedic surgery. Ann Rheum Dis 2001;60:214–7.

22. Sany J, Anaya JM, Canovas F, et al. Influence of methotrexate on the frequency of postoperative infectious complications in patients with rheumatoid arthritis. J Rheumatol 1993;20:1129–32.

23. Jain A, Witbreuk M, Ball C, et al. Influence of steroids and methotrexate on wound complications after elective rheumatoid hand and wrist surgery. J Hand Surg Am 2002;27:449–55.

24. Bongartz T. Elective orthopedic surgery and perioperative DMARD management: many questions, fewer answers, and some opinions. J Rheumatol 2007;34:653–5.

25. Goupille P, Pham T, Sibilia J, et al. Perioperative management of patients with rheumatoid arthritis treated with TNF-alpha blocking agents. Semin Arthritis Rheum 2007;37:202–3.

26. Scanzello CR, Figgie MP, Nestor BJ, et al. Perioperative management of medications used in the treatment of rheumatoid arthritis. HSS J 2006;2:141–7.

27. Capobianco CM, Ramanujam CL, Zgonis T. Rheumatoid Foot and Ankle Surgery. Curr Rheumatol Rev 2010;6:77–86.

28. Forestier R, André-Vert J, Guillez P, et al. Non-drug treatment (excluding surgery) in rheumatoid arthritis: clinical practice guidelines. Joint Bone Spine 2009;76: 691–8.

29. Löfkvist UB, Brattström M, Geborek P, et al. Individually adapted lightweight walking aids with moulded handles for patients with severely deforming chronic arthritis. Scand J Rheumatol 1988;17:167–73.

30. Wickman AM, Pinzur MS, Kadanoff R. Health-related quality of life for patients with rheumatoid arthritis foot involvement. Foot Ankle Int 2004;25:19–26.

Perioperative Management of the Dysvascular Foot and Ankle

Crystal L. Ramanujam, DPM, Zacharia Facaros, DPM, Thomas Zgonis, DPM*

KEYWORDS

- Peripheral vascular disease • Foot surgery • Toe pressure
- Angiography • Diabetes

Foot and ankle surgery in patients with peripheral vascular disease (PVD) requires special considerations to produce optimal outcomes. Atherosclerosis is the main risk factor for PVD, yet most people affected are asymptomatic. Approximately 20% of the general population older than 55 years have chronic atherosclerotic lower extremity disease.[1] Only about 20% of these patients present to a health care professional due to symptoms, and another 20% do not seek medical care despite the presence of symptoms. The most common symptom of PVD is intermittent claudication, and according to Nolan and colleagues,[2] approximately 25% of the symptomatic patients under medical care develop progressive symptoms within 5 years, 5% to 10% require surgical intervention, and 1% to 2% undergo major amputation.

Several patients presenting for a specific foot or ankle problem have previously undiagnosed PVD, and in many cases, a thorough workup by a foot and ankle specialist can determine the extent of the disease. The diagnosis of significant PVD may not necessarily preclude foot or ankle surgery; however, its finding may alter procedural timing, procedure selection, and postoperative course. In emergent situations such as limb- or life-threatening infection, patients may proceed to surgery immediately, because in these cases, infection supersedes vascular status. Whether the patient is undergoing an elective or urgent procedure, careful attention to appropriate perioperative management by the entire surgical team can prevent disastrous complications.

Division of Podiatric Medicine and Surgery, Department of Orthopaedics, University of Texas Health Science Center at San Antonio, San Antonio, TX, USA
* Corresponding author.
E-mail address: Zgonis@uthscsa.edu

Perioperative Nursing Clinics 6 (2011) 17–26
doi:10.1016/j.cpen.2010.10.003
periopnursing.theclinics.com
1556-7931/11/$ – see front matter © 2011 Elsevier Inc. All rights reserved.

PREOPERATIVE WORKUP

In any case, a thorough history must be taken to identify possible predisposition for PVD. Advanced age, cigarette smoking, abnormal glucose tolerance, hyperlipidemia, and hypertension are among the most common risk factors for arteriocclusive disease.[3] Furthermore, increased plasma fibrinogen levels,[4] hyperhomocysteinemia,[5,6] and high-sensitivity C-reactive protein[7] also increase risk of PVD. The presence of more than 1 risk factor leads to a cumulative risk that is even greater than their additive risks. Patients should be counseled regarding modifiable risk factors such as smoking, and every effort at reduction or cessation should be attempted when considering an elective foot or ankle procedure. Before any surgery, a thorough, interactive discussion between the surgeon and patient must be undertaken regarding all risks, complications, and alternatives to surgical treatment, especially in relation to PVD. Possibilities and questions should be raised regarding risks of minor or major amputation in situations attempting limb salvage.

Physical examination can be used as a screening tool but is not 100% reliable for diagnosis of PVD. As stated before, intermittent claudication is the most common presenting symptom. It is demonstrated as cramping or fatigue in one or both lower extremities that is reproducible upon walking a specific distance and is relieved by several minutes of rest. The anatomic location of claudication often predicts the level of occlusive disease: symptoms in the calf muscles indicate infrainguinal disease, whereas those occurring in the buttocks or thighs indicate aortoiliac disease.[8] Diminished or absent peripheral pulses may also be an indicator but often depends on the specific level. Palpation of pulses should be attempted from the abdominal aorta to the foot, with auscultation for bruits in the abdominal and pelvic regions. A handheld Doppler probe is a useful tool for initial examination if pulses are not readily palpable. Athough an abnormal femoral pulse has a high specificity and positive predictive value, it comprises a low sensitivity for large vessel disease.[9] Absence of the dorsalis pedis pulse may be a normal anatomic variant, noted in approximately 10% of the population. The best single discriminator for PVD in the physical examination is an abnormal posterior tibial pulse. Other possible clinical findings include lack of pedal hair growth, delayed capillary refill, cool skin or abnormal temperature gradient, pallor on elevation of the limb with dependent rubor, skin atrophy, cyanosis of the toes, nonhealing ulceration, and necrotic tissue. Plain film radiography can provide clues of PVD by demonstrating calcified vessels at the lower extremity; however, this is not a reliable measure of the extent of disease because patients showing vessel calcification may still have adequate distal perfusion.

A high index of suspicion based on history and physical examination findings should lead the health care provider to further noninvasive testing to define the level and extent of arterial occlusive disease. Routine screening laboratory studies can evaluate for associated systemic risk factors and contributing issues: complete blood count may indicate presence of hematologic diseases, fasting blood glucose may reveal the possibility of diabetes, lipid profiles may indicate hyperlipidemia, coagulation studies may uncover thrombotic disease, and serum homocysteine levels help screen for hyperhomocysteinemia.

Full lower-extremity noninvasive examination is warranted when considering foot and ankle surgery for a patient with PVD to determine healing potential. This testing includes ankle-brachial index (ABI), toe-brachial index (TBI), segmental limb pressures, segmental volume plethysmography also known as pulse-volume recording (PVR), and transcutaneous oxygen pressure (TcPO2). ABI and TBI are simple and relatively inexpensive methods performed by measuring the resting systolic blood pressures in the ankle or toe in relation to that of the arm; the value resulting from dividing the distal pressure by that of the arm provides a measure of the severity of PVD (**Table 1**). Care should be taken when interpreting these values because vessel calcification can lead to false elevation. Raue and colleagues[10] found a significantly higher percentage of calcifications in the region of the abdominal aorta, the iliac, and the peripheral arteries of the legs in persons with PVD.

Segmental limb pressures are assessed by placement of blood pressure cuffs at different levels of the lower extremity. A finding of 20 mm Hg or greater reduction in pressure is considered significant if such a gradient is found between segments along the same extremity or when compared with the same level in the contralateral limb. Segmental volume plethysmography or PVR is often used with segmental pressures to determine the level of arterial disease. These measurements are conducted by injecting a standard volume of air into pneumatic cuffs placed at different levels of the lower extremity. Volume changes in the limb segment below the cuff are translated into pulsatile pressure, which is detected by a transducer and then displayed as a pressure pulse contour.[11] A normal PVR is defined as a systolic upstroke with a sharp systolic peak followed by a downstroke that contains a prominent dicrotic notch. A change in the PVR indicates proximal arterial obstruction and is due to the dissipated energy that occurs from arterial narrowing.[12] TcPO2 is defined as the pressure at which skin perfusion returns as an inflated blood pressure cuff is slowly deflated. This test is helpful for determining healing potential, selecting amputation level, evaluating revascularization procedures, and assessing progression of PVD. Traditionally, TcPO2 values greater than 40 mm Hg are associated with good healing, between 20 and 40 mm Hg with intermediate healing, and less than 20 mm Hg with poor healing.[13] Individual studies by Ladurner and colleagues[14] and Ruangsetakit and colleagues[15] both found that diabetic foot wounds associated with a TcPO2 reading less than 20 mm Hg demonstrated a significantly decreased probability of healing compared with those associated with a TcPO2 greater than 40 mm Hg.

Duplex Doppler ultrasonography examination of the lower extremity starts at the common femoral artery and proceeds distally to the popliteal artery; the normal peripheral arterial velocity waveform demonstrates a triphasic pattern. Koelemay and colleagues[16] performed a meta-analysis that found that sensitivity and specificity of this technique for more than 50% stenoses or occlusions were 86% and 97% for aortoiliac disease and 80% and 98% for femoropopliteal disease.

Based on the results of noninvasive testing, a formal consultation to a vascular surgeon may be warranted before definitive foot and ankle surgery. The vascular team can perform conventional diagnostic angiography to accurately determine the site and severity of stenosis or occlusion. Digital subtraction angiography (DSA) still remains the gold-standard arterial imaging study used in the diagnosis of PVD

Table 1
ABI as an indicator of PVD

ABI Value	Degree of Arterial Compromise	Action
Above 1.2	Noncompressible calcification	Refer routinely
1.0–1.2	Normal	None
0.9–1.0	Acceptable	
0.8–0.9	Some disease	Manage risk factors
0.4–0.8	Moderate disease (multilevel occlusion)	Routine referral to vascular specialist
<0.4	Severe disease (multilevel occlusion)	Urgent referral to vascular specialist

(**Fig. 1**). However, this test is usually reserved for when an intervention (either endovascular or traditional open surgery) is planned. This technique is considered the most accurate, because it can reveal stenosis, dilatation, occlusion, plaque ulceration, or thrombotic material. DSA is the most commonly used method of assessing the arteries before surgery but possesses one major disadvantage compared with the other techniques, because it requires the placement of a needle in the artery.[17] This can be uncomfortable, but it is the only method of assessment that can also be used to treat arterial disease by angioplasty.

Magnetic resonance angiography (MRA) is one of the newer techniques that relies on powerful magnets to align water molecules in the body tissues but is technically challenging to execute (**Fig. 2**). It is a painless and fairly rapid form of assessment but is noisy and some patients feel claustrophobic during the procedure. MRA can be used to assess almost any artery in the body but found particularly useful in the assessment of carotid artery disease. It does not require puncture of an artery and consequently is only useful in the diagnosis of disease and cannot be used to treat arterial problems. MRA has been shown to be more sensitive than DSA at times; however, spatial resolution has been found to be inferior.[18] As with any advanced imaging involving contrast injection, there is a risk of kidney damage in some patients.[19]

Computed tomography angiography (CTA) uses X rays to produce horizontal cross-sectional images through the body, which are then reconstructed using computers to produce longitudinal and 3-dimensional images. The advantage of CTA is that it does not require a puncture of an artery, although as with MRA, if an angioplasty is required, CTA must be performed separately using conventional angiography. Contrast medium is also required in this type of imaging. CTA is becoming more popular and newer imaging suites are able to combine cross-sectional CT images with angiography in 3 dimensions. CTA offers a wide and diverse range of applications in

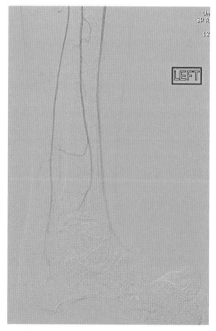

Fig. 1. DSA illustrating runoff at the anterior tibial, posterior tibial, and peroneal arteries in a diabetic man with nonhealing open wound and osteomyelitis of the forefoot.

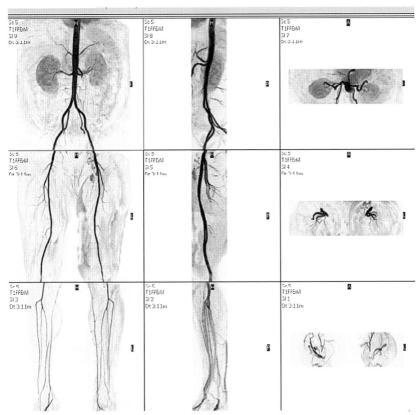

Fig. 2. MRA shows vascular patency from the abdominal aorta to the lower extremities in a patient with PVD with significant hindfoot arthrosis being considered for elective arthrodesis procedures.

the evaluation of the lower extremity arterial system.[20] Furthermore, carbon dioxide (CO_2) is used as an alternate angiographic contrast agent that can be delivered through a hand injection or a pump. Because the use of CO_2 is not associated with nephrotoxicity or allergic reactions, it is increasingly being used as a contrast agent for arteriography.[21,22]

Decision for the type and extent of required vascular surgical intervention is made based on the patient's symptoms and medical history, physical findings, noninvasive testing, and diagnostic imaging. When conservative therapy fails, endovascular procedures may be effective, particularly if the disease extent is minimal. Endovascular procedure, or repair from within a blood vessel, has gained popularity over recent years because of several distinct advantages offered over open surgical revascularization for selected lesions.[23] This procedure is performed with local anesthesia, enabling the treatment of patients who are at high risk for general anesthesia. Furthermore, the morbidity and mortality associated is low compared with open surgical revascularization. After successful percutaneous revascularization, patients are ambulatory on the day of treatment and can often return to normal activity within 24 to 48 hours of an uncomplicated procedure. Moreover, endovascular therapies generally do not preclude or alter subsequent surgery and may be repeated if necessary. Techniques executed for endovascular therapy include percutaneous transluminal angioplasty (PTA) with or without stents, using bare, drug-eluting, or covered stents; subintimal angioplasty; cutting balloon PTA; cryoplasty; brachytherapy; laser angioplasty; atherectomy; and percutaneous bypass.[23]

Although endovascular options for treating peripheral arterial disease continue to expand and outcomes continue to improve, open surgery may be considered for selected patients with claudication who fail endovascular therapy or are not candidates for it. Patients with more severe symptoms typically have more extensive disease that is treated best with open surgery or with a combination of open and endovascular therapies. Open surgical revascularization is warranted for patients with complex lesions that are not amenable to catheter-based intervention, as well as being favored in younger patients with prolonged life expectancy who require a more durable revascularization. Furthermore, open surgery is the optimal revascularization strategy for patients who are relatively fit and can withstand the rigors of an open procedure. The standard open procedure is bypass grafting with or without femoral endarterectomy, with or without adjunctive inflow treatment.[24] The preferred graft conduit for infrainguinal bypass is autogenous saphenous vein, but other autogenous venous conduits may be harvested. The inflow artery must have uncompromised hemodynamics, and arterial outflow should be continuous to the ankle and foot. Other significant variables are vein graft origin, graft diameter, and graft length, all of which are influential toward short-term and long-term patencies.[24]

An inpatient observation period is usually required after endovascular or open procedures for prevention and treatment of complications, with the duration of hospital stay depending on the procedure performed. The foot and ankle surgeon must coordinate timing of their surgical procedures based on direct recommendations from the vascular specialist. Because ambulation with the assistance of a physical therapist usually starts gradually on the first or second postoperative day after bypass procedures, immediate secondary foot procedures should be delayed. Several procedures such as debridement or distal amputation can be performed during the same hospital stay, whereas more extensive reconstructive procedures should be performed once the patient has fully recovered from the revascularization and has been deemed as having optimal lower extremity perfusion to support healing of the foot and ankle procedures. Knowledge of medications relating to revascularization, such as patients who may be on antiplatelet or other anticoagulation therapy, is necessary to discontinue or bridge patients before elective foot and ankle procedures to limit blood loss and to ensure safety.

INTRAOPERATIVE MANAGEMENT

Operating room setup has important implications for the patient with PVD. Appropriate positioning of the patient and padding of bony prominences must be addressed for the duration of the operative episode. Handling of the patient should also be careful and deliberate to avoid excessive pressure to the skin. Tourniquet use is usually contraindicated in patients with severe PVD, because use of this device can cause increased risk of further stenosis. In addition, tourniquet use directly over the site of revascularization is usually avoided if possible during foot and ankle surgeries in patients who have undergone vascular procedures such as arterial bypass within the last 6 months. In extensive reconstructive procedures, such as those involving the Charcot foot and ankle, a tourniquet or a compressive bandage may be used with permission from the vascular surgeon after revascularization for a very short duration to provide a bloodless field during careful dissection for visualization and hardware placement.

For patients with PVD, choices regarding incisional approaches should be mindful of local vasculature based on the 6 angiosomes supplied by the 3 main arteries and their branches in the foot and ankle.[25] Special attention to atraumatic technique by both the surgeon and assistants is imperative in these patients, regardless of whether or not they have undergone revascularization procedures. Careful tissue handling during dissection, retraction, and hardware placement can avoid detrimental complications. Suture techniques to avoid tension at skin margins and underlying tissue is a must in patients with PVD. If excessive tension is apparent as evidenced by pallor appearance of the skin upon closure of an incision, methods to reduce the tension such as pie-crusting or fenestration techniques can be performed to allow relaxation and local hyperemia. Likewise, dressings placed on the operative limb should avoid constriction or excessive pressure against the surgical site and surrounding skin. Pressure necrosis can lead to ulceration and infection in areas that previously had no problems. Cast or splint application may only be used when absolutely necessary in patients with severe PVD; instead, bulky gauze dressings and a simple postoperative shoe may be the best option depending on the procedure and level of patient compliance. Use of external fixation to facilitate off-loading has been described for use in selected patients even after revascularization.

POSTOPERATIVE CARE AND REHABILITATION

Observation in the postoperative period is imperative, because immediate treatment for any evidence of ischemia should be instituted. The importance of careful dressing application cannot be overemphasized as many complications in patients with PVD undergoing foot and ankle surgery are iatrogenically induced. Dressing coverings that contain elastic materials should be avoided, because excessive compression at the foot with these materials is common. Immobilization options are based on the type of foot or ankle surgery as well as any type of revascularization that has been performed. For patients who have undergone revascularization, ambulation is encouraged; therefore, this can be a challenge when the patient has also undergone a foot procedure requiring non–weight-bearing status. Physical therapy for crutch and/or walker training to maintain non–weight bearing to the operative limb is required. The use of newer assistive devices such as specialized rolling walkers can facilitate mobility in these patients.

Appropriate precautions should be taken for patients with PVD who may be sedentary or require bed rest after a reconstructive foot or ankle procedure; this includes adequate anticoagulation therapy and use of off-loading modalities to prevent decubitus ulcerations. Off-loading boots for protection of the heels, frequent changes in position within the bed through assistance from nursing, and the use of pressure-reducing mattresses or beds should be considered. For patients with compromised distal perfusion and who have undergone elective foot or ankle surgery, caregivers should abstain from the use of ice or other local cooling devices. For the same reason, excessive elevation of the foot or any position that may limit circulation should also be avoided.

Infection is a risk for any surgical procedure but can be especially challenging in the patient afflicted with PVD. Macrovascular and microvascular diseases can affect the bioavailability and effectiveness of systemic antibiotics. Local antibiotic delivery systems, such as antibiotic-impregnated cement beads or spacers, may be a good option in such patients to allow for increased local levels of antibiotic for resolution

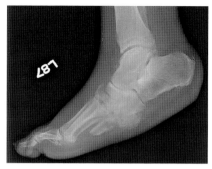

Fig. 3. Lateral foot radiograph demonstrating extensive midfoot Charcot neuroarthropathy in patient after undergoing partial ray amputations and revascularization via lower extremity bypass.

of infection. Dysvascular tissue at the foot or ankle is more prone to infection; therefore early signs of ischemia or necrosis should alert the health care provider to provide aggressive treatment. Hyperbaric oxygen therapy can be a useful adjunct to local wound care in selected patients.

Smoking in the postoperative period can be detrimental to surgical outcomes in the foot and ankle even for patients without PVD, yet the effect is compounded in patients with PVD. Smoking has been shown to adversely affect wound healing.[26] In addition, lower rates of osteotomy union, bony fusion, and higher rates of postoperative infection for foot and ankle procedures have been found in smokers. Consequently, formal counseling on cessation should be initiated in the preoperative setting and continued throughout the healing process.[27,28]

Specific postoperative complications relating to revascularization procedures include early postoperative occlusion, hemorrhagic problems, graft infection, cardiac morbidity, and restenosis. Special considerations should be directed toward protecting the foot and ankle in patients who have undergone revascularizations, because there is a risk for development of Charcot neuroarthropathy.[29] In the neuropathic extremity, the resultant hyperemic response after revascularization of the extremity is thought to contribute to increased osteoclastic activity with subsequent osteolysis and joint collapse. Surgically induced Charcot neuroarthropathy after amputation of a digit or partial ray of the foot is also a concern in diabetic patients (**Fig. 3**).[30] The use of extra depth shoes, bracing, and custom inlays with fillers for amputation sites as indicated can facilitate stabilization of the foot, as well as redistribute pressure at bony deformities to decrease risk of ulceration.

SUMMARY

Thorough knowledge and skills in the appropriate workup and care of the patient with PVD is essential when executing foot and ankle surgery. Advances in medical technology, wound care, and surgical techniques have given health care providers further options for reconstruction and limb salvage. Despite these developments, preventive treatment continues to be foremost in reducing complications. The entire surgical team should have a firm grasp of the risks involved with treating patients with PVD undergoing urgent, emergent, or elective foot and ankle surgery. From the initial evaluation of the patient to the operative setting and throughout the recovery period, each step in treatment has direct impact on outcomes in this high-risk population.

REFERENCES

1. Hankey GJ, Norman PE, Eikelboom JW. Medical treatment of peripheral arterial disease. JAMA 2006;295:547–53.
2. Nolan B, Finlayson S, Tosteson A, et al. The treatment of disabling intermittent claudication in patients with superficial femoral artery occlusive disease–decision analysis. J Vasc Surg 2007;45:1179–84.
3. Chi YW, Jaff MR. Optimal risk factor modification and medical management of the patient with peripheral arterial disease. Catheter Cardiovasc Interv 2008;71:475–89.
4. Daskalopoulou SS, Pathmarajah M, Kakkos SK, et al. Association between ankle - brachial index and risk factor profile in patients newly diagnosed with intermittent claudication. Circ J 2008;72:441–8.
5. Garofolo L, Barros N Jr, Miranda F Jr, et al. Association of increased levels of homocysteine and peripheral arterial disease in a Japanese-Brazilian population. Eur J Vasc Endovasc Surg 2007;34:23–8.
6. Taute BM, Taute R, Heins S, et al. Hyperhomocysteinemia: marker of systemic atherosclerosis in peripheral arterial disease. Int Angiol 2004;23:35–40.
7. Pradhan AD, Shrivastava S, Cook NR, et al. Symptomatic peripheral arterial disease in women: nontraditional biomarkers of elevated risk. Circulation 2008; 117:823–31.
8. Cournot M, Boccalon H, Cambou JP, et al. Accuracy of the screening physical examination to identify subclinical atherosclerosis and peripheral arterial disease in asymptomatic subjects. J Vasc Surg 2007;46:1215–21.
9. Criqui MH, Fronek A, Klauber MR, et al. The sensitivity, specificity, and predictive value of traditional clinical evaluation of peripheral arterial disease: results from noninvasive testing in a defined population. Circulation 1985;71:516–22.
10. Raue I, Sauer I, Voigt H. Cardiac findings and vascular calcification in arteriosclerotic obstructive disease in the pelvis and leg region. Z Gesamte Inn Med 1980;35:166–9.
11. Kempczinski RF. Segmental volume plethysmography in the diagnosis of lower extremity arterial occlusive disease. J Cardiovasc Surg 1982;23:125–9.
12. Darling RC, Raines JK, Brener BJ, et al. Quantitative segmental pulse volume recorder: a clinical tool. Surgery 1972;72:873–7.
13. Wyss CR, Harrington RM, Burgess EM, et al. Transcutaneous oxygen tension as a predictor of success after an amputation. J Bone Joint Surg Am 1988;70:203–7.
14. Ladurner R, Küper M, Königsrainer I, et al. Predictive value of routine transcutaneous tissue oxygen tension (tcpO2) measurement for the risk of non-healing and amputation in diabetic foot ulcer patients with non-palpable pedal pulses. Med Sci Monit 2010;16:273–7.
15. Ruangsetakit C, Chinsakchai K, Mahawongkajit P, et al. Transcutaneous oxygen tension: a useful predictor of ulcer healing in critical limb ischaemia. J Wound Care 2010;19:202–6.
16. Koelemay MJ, den Hartog D, Prins MH, et al. Diagnosis of arterial disease of the lower extremities with duplex ultrasonography. Br J Surg 1996;83:404.
17. White C. Clinical practice: intermittent claudication. N Engl J Med 2007;356: 1241–50.
18. Pomposelli F. Arterial imaging in patients with lower extremity ischemia and diabetes mellitus. J Vasc Surg 2010;52(Suppl 3):81–91.
19. Detrenis S, Meschi M, del Mar Jordana Sanchez M, et al. Contrast medium induced nephropathy in urological practice. J Urol 2007;178:1164–70.
20. Foley WD, Stonely T. CT angiography of the lower extremities. Radiol Clin North Am 2010;48:367–96.

21. Kerns SR, Hawkins IF Jr. Carbon dioxide digital subtraction angiography: expanding applications and technical evolution. Am J Roentgenol 1995;164:735–41.

22. Hawkins IF, Cho KJ, Caridi JG. Carbon dioxide in angiography to reduce the risk of contrast-induced nephropathy. Radiol Clin North Am 2009;47:813–25.

23. White CJ, Gray WA. Endovascular therapies for peripheral arterial disease: an evidence-based review. Circulation 2007;116:2203–15.

24. Schanzer A, Conte MS. Critical limb ischemia. Curr Treat Options Cardiovasc Med 2010;12:214–29.

25. Attinger CE, Evans KK, Bulan E, et al. Angiosomes of the foot and ankle and clinical implications for limb salvage: reconstruction, incisions, and revascularization. Plast Reconstr Surg 2006;117(Suppl 7):261–93.

26. Haverstock BD, Mandracchia VJ. Cigarette smoking and bone healing: implications in foot and ankle surgery. J Foot Ankle Surg 1998;37:69–74.

27. Marx RC, Mizel MS. What's new in foot and ankle surgery. J Bone Joint Surg Am 2010;92:512–23.

28. Walker NM, Morris SA, Cannon LB. The effect of pre-operative counseling on smoking patterns in patients undergoing forefoot surgery. Foot Ankle Surg 2009;15:86–9.

29. Edelman SV, Kosofsky EM, Paul RA, et al. Neuro-osteoarthropathy (Charcot's joints) in diabetes mellitus following revascularization surgery: three case reports and a review of the literature. Arch Intern Med 1987;147:1504–8.

30. Zgonis T, Stapleton JJ, Shibuya N, et al. Surgically induced charcot neuroarthropathy following partial forefoot amputation in diabetes. J Wound Care 2007;16:57–9.

Urgent and Emergent Foot and Ankle Infections

Claire M. Capobianco, DPM[a],*, Shirmeen Lakhani, DPM[b]

KEYWORDS

- Diabetes • Foot • Infections • Necrotizing fasciitis • Surgery

Foot and ankle infections that necessitate operative intervention warrant appropriate attention from the entire operative team. Because the foot is a highly complicated weight-bearing structure consisting of 4 layers of musculature, 9 compartments, 28 bones, intertriginous areas and areas of minimal soft tissue coverage, infections can be multifarious in nature, develop insidiously, and spread quickly via extrinsic or fascial conduits. Surgical decompression is crucial for the management of urgent and emergent infections; thus, the most common causes, surgical management and anesthesia, and nursing considerations are reviewed.

ABSCESSES

Abscess formation in the foot and ankle warrants urgent surgical management. Because the plantar foot has multiple fascial compartments and layers of muscula-ture, plantar abscesses are often far more extensive than they might appear. In addi-tion, infected fluids may progress along paths of least resistance, such as tendon sheaths or fascial planes, and not uncommonly may extend to the level of the ankle or further proximally. On surgical exploration, violation of deeper soft-tissue struc-tures, such as tendons, capsules, and joints, may indicate more aggressive or insid-ious spread. In these cases especially, evaluation of adjacent osseous structures for signs of osteomyelitis is crucial. Preoperative radiography and intraoperative biopsy and culture may confirm the diagnosis of osteomyelitis, the importance of which cannot be underscored. Depending on the location and extent, the confirmed presence of osteomyelitis alters both the surgical and medical management approaches and may result in prolonged administration of parenteral antibiotics, addi-tional osseous debridement, staged reconstructive procedures, or even amputation **(Fig. 1)**.

[a] Orthopaedic Associates of Southern Delaware, 17005 Old Orchard Road, Lewes, DE 19958, USA
[b] Division of Podiatric Medicine and Surgery, Department of Orthopaedics, University of Texas Health Science Center at San Antonio, 7703 Floyd Curl Drive, San Antonio, TX 78829, USA
* Corresponding author.
E-mail address: coatescm@gmail.com

Perioperative Nursing Clinics 6 (2011) 27–33
doi:10.1016/j.cpen.2010.10.005
1556-7931/11/$ – see front matter © 2011 Elsevier Inc. All rights reserved.

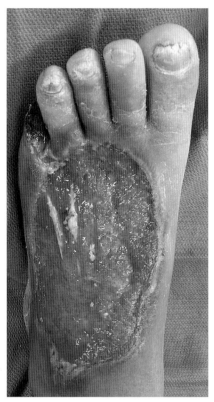

Fig. 1. The left foot after an aggressive surgical debridement of the dorsal aspect from an infected left fifth digit.

PUNCTURE WOUNDS

Puncture wounds to the plantar aspect of the foot deserve additional attention because these wounds may deteriorate into urgent or emergent infections via abscess formation in deep compartments. The incidence of serious complications following plantar puncture wound has been reported to be 2% to 10%.[1,2] The location of the puncture wound is important. The foot is divided into 3 zones: (1) distal to the submetatarsal neck region, (2) the plantar arch, and (3) the plantar heel. Zones 1 and 3 are at the highest risk for development of osteomyelitis and septic arthritis.[1] A retained foreign body nidus has been implicated in severe infections following puncture wounds that ultimately require surgery.[2,3] The morbidity following puncture wounds is significantly greater in patients with diabetes and is associated with a 46-fold increased likelihood of subsequent amputation.[4] Wounds that result from punctures through tennis shoes and socks most commonly involve *Pseudomonas aeruginosa*. Other organisms common to initial wound infection include *Staphylococcus aureus* and group A *Streptococcus*.[2]

DIABETIC FOOT AND ANKLE INFECTIONS

Serious diabetes mellitus–associated foot infections are common and may involve ulceration, puncture, abscess, necrotizing fasciitis, and/or osteomyelitis. Metabolic instability may also present concurrently, which significantly complicates the treatment algorithm.

Some investigators cite that, in the diabetic population specifically, infected foot wounds are responsible for a quarter of all diabetes-related admissions in Great Britain and the United States.[4] Although the overall management and surgical approaches to the diabetic foot are beyond the scope of this article, it is widely known that poor glycemic control confers a host of end-organ manifestations, including retinopathy, nephropathy, vasculopathy, immunocompromise, and peripheral neuropathy. Neuropathy paired with improper or ill-fitting shoe gear, poor hygiene, or maladaptive habits such as walking barefoot or excessive activity frequently result in silent ulceration or puncture wounds. These wounds may become severely infected secondary to inadequate leukocyte phagocytosis of bacteria in the setting of hyperglycemia. Significant hyperglycemia may also result in diabetic ketoacidosis and electrolyte instability on presentation to the emergency department. The risk-benefit analysis of surgical decompression timing in the setting of metabolic instability, underlying end-organ abnormality, and emergent infection is of utmost importance, and communication between multidisciplinary specialists is crucial.

The statistics about diabetes and foot infections are sobering. Diabetic patients have an approximately 25% risk of developing a pedal complication over the course of their lifetime.[5] A significant proportion of these wounds become infected and affect soft tissue, deep structures, and/or bone. The literature indicates a wide variety in the prevalence of underlying bone infection in patients with diabetic ulcerations, depending on the cohort of patients studied. Crucially, diabetic patients with severe-enough foot infections to warrant emergent or surgical care have up to a 66% likelihood of underlying osteomyelitis.[6] Chronic pedal ulcerations are the primary risk factor for development of contiguous osteomyelitis,[7] and, as a result, factors that delay wound healing (hyperglycemia, insufficient offloading, peripheral arterial disease, osseous instability, overactivity) increase the incidence of osteomyelitis. Consequently, severe diabetic foot infections have been reported to confer a 25% risk of major amputation on an already high-risk patient population (**Fig. 2**).[8]

In diabetic patients, severe soft tissue infections tend to be polymicrobial in nature, including mixed gram-positive and gram-negative aerobic and anaerobic bacteria and occasionally fungus.[9–12] In diabetic osteomyelitis, the organisms most frequently isolated include *S aureus*, *Streptococci*, coagulase-negative *Staphylococci*, *Escherichia*

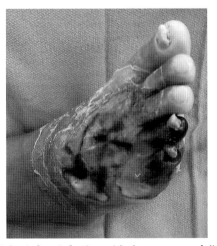

Fig. 2. A severe initial diabetic foot infection with the presence of distal forefoot gangrene.

coli, *Klebsiella pneumonia*, the *Proteus* species, *Pseudomonas aeruginosa*, and anaerobes (notably the *Peptococci*). In addition, bacteria that were long considered as normal skin contaminants (*Corynebacterium* species and coagulase-negative staphylococci) have been cultured from osteomyelitic bone in reports on diabetic patients.[13,14] Experts postulate that in an immunocompromised host, the actuality of these species as true pathogens does conditionally exist in the absence of intraoperative wound specimen contamination; a concordant microscopic diagnosis of osteomyelitis further strengthens the evidence.[12,15,16] To further complicate matters, an increasing presence of resistant bacteria, including methicillin-resistant *S aureus*,[10,11,17–19] vancomycin-resistant *S aureus*,[20] and extended-spectrum β-lactamase gram-negative bacilli with multidrug resistance,[21] has been reported in the literature on the diabetic foot. Accuracy in subsequent antibiotic management rests on proper intraoperative bone and soft tissue biopsies for the most precise identification of the causative pathogens.[16]

In the foot and ankle, severe infections limited to soft tissue can be devastating and can result in a significant loss of crucial plantar adipose tissue and musculotendinous functionality. Furthermore, when osteomyelitis affects the underlying bony architecture, debridement and partial amputations predictably affect the resultant biomechanics of the residual limb. In the past, many of these limbs were considered unsalvageable and were amputated. Controversy exists regarding antibiotic management in diabetic foot osteomyelitis and therapy ought to be tailored in a patient-specific fashion. Often, functional amputation of the affected bone paired with a limited parenteral and prolonged oral regimen is recommended. In the setting of adequate perfusion, new approaches, advances in surgical techniques, and staged orthoplastic procedures have restored previously unsalvageable distal lower extremities. The importance of limb salvage in the diabetic population cannot be understated because approximately 50% of patients undergoing a major limb amputation become bilateral amputees within 2 to 5 years or suffer a major cardiovascular event.[22,23]

NECROTIZING FASCIITIS

Although uncommon, necrotizing fasciitis of the foot and lower extremity is a surgical emergency. Clinically, necrotizing fasciitis may appear as an edematous, often fluctuant, progressively worsening area with mottled overlying skin, ecchymoses or petechiae. Skin color changes from erythematous to violaceous to cyanotic. Conversely, rapid progression of erythema to overt gangrene may present.[12] Lymphangiitis may or may not be present. Marked leukocytosis, hyponatremia, pain out of proportion, and systemic symptoms present in the sensate patient, but neuropathic diabetic patients may lack some or all of these symptoms.[12] The infection spreads rapidly along fascial planes and, indeed, is truly only diagnosable with an intraoperative culture, fascial biopsy, and histopathologic analysis. As initially described in 1952, the infectious process results in massive necrosis of fascia and subcutaneous tissue, with relative sparing of the underlying muscle,[24] but severe variants may involve underlying muscle necrosis in the lower extremities in synergic necrotizing cellulitis.[12]

The so-called flesh-eating bacteria that causes necrotizing fasciitis is actually more than 1 species. Necrotizing fasciitis may present in 1 of 2 common patterns; type 1 is caused by polymicrobial infection, and type 2 by streptococcal (usually group A) with possible concurrent staphylococcal infection. Intravenous drug use, obesity, and alcoholism are predisposing factors for type 1. Diabetes or immunocompromise are major predisposing factors for both type 1 and type 2 presentations.[24] A rare variant of necrotizing fasciitis may be a symptom of septicemia of the marine-related organism *Vibrio vulnificus*.[25] Regardless of the cause, the definitive management of these patients involves emergent surgical decompression and debridement of all nonviable tissue, appropriate parenteral antibiotic therapy, medical optimization, repeated irrigation and debridement, and staged reconstruction of the lower extremity. The overall impact of necrotizing fasciitis is significant, with an estimate of mortality of 25%[24] and, in diabetic patients, a 50% likelihood of subsequent major amputation.[26]

ANESTHESIA AND PERIOPERATIVE NURSING CONSIDERATIONS

In the sensate patient with an urgent foot and ankle infection, general or spinal anesthesia is warranted to facilitate adequate debridement of all necrotic tissue and exploration and evacuation of all affected compartments and purulence. In the diabetic patient, serious infections may be complicated by ketoacidosis and metabolic instability. In urgent infections, severe hyperglycemia and electrolyte imbalances ought to be stabilized expediently by the medical team before operative intervention. Conversely, surgical decompression may be necessary emergently to treat or prevent blossoming sepsis, especially in necrotizing fasciitis.

Serious infection spurs increased metabolic demand, which can stress an already diseased heart. Diabetes predisposes patients to both atherosclerotic cardiac disease and cardiomyopathy and thus doubles to triples the perioperative morbidity and mortality risk.[27] Elevated glycosylated hemoglobin values are associated with diabetic cardiomyopathy, retinopathy, and nephropathy. In addition, with anesthesia, cardiac autonomic neuropathy precipitates more hemodynamic instability and a greater need for vasoactive medications during surgery.[27] Diabetic patients are also known to have an impaired hypoxic ventilatory drive response and are at a greater risk for intraoperative hypothermia.[27] Newer antidiabetic medications, such as the amylin analogue pramlintide and incretin peptide exenatide, function by delaying gastric emptying time to reduce postprandial serum glucose; these effects may be additive to underlying autonomic gastroparesis and must also be accounted for in diabetic patients undergoing surgery.[28]

The prevalence of peripheral arterial disease is also 4 times greater in patients with diabetes than in the nondiabetic population.[4] In urgent-emergent infections, frequently more than 1 fascial compartment is violated and, as previously discussed, general or spinal anesthesia is desired. In patients with dense peripheral neuropathy and superficial or limited infectious margins, local or regional anesthesia may be appropriate. Any use of local anesthesia must be carefully considered because the acidic pH of the infected tissue predictably impairs the effectiveness and may result in inadequate anesthesia.

Specific nursing considerations in the management of patients with foot infections revolve around careful monitoring of the high-risk patient and accuracy in labeling intraoperative specimens. Proper and expeditious handling of specimens is paramount to diagnosis and further management of the patient, especially when multiple bone and soft tissue samples are obtained. The need for narcotic pain medications postoperatively in patients with diabetic neuropathy must also be carefully considered, especially if the decompressed area extends beyond the distribution of neuropathy. Because anemia of chronic disease is common in the diabetic patient, intraoperative blood loss and/or inadequate volume expansion may exacerbate orthostatic hypotension, weakness, or lethargy. Wanton postoperative elevation of lower extremities may impair the already marginal perfusion in the patient with peripheral arterial disease, so caution must be exercised at the discretion of the surgeon.

SUMMARY

Abscess formation must be considered in the differential diagnosis for patients with erythema and edema that does not improve with elevation of the affected extremity. In the diabetic and immunocompromised populations especially, urgent foot and ankle infections may present insidiously and progress rapidly. Optimization during the perioperative period for these higher-risk patients depends on careful monitoring and effective communication within a multidisciplinary team. In general, broad-spectrum antibiotic coverage, appropriate anesthesia selection, adequate surgical decompression and debridement, and, sometimes, staged surgical intervention are integral to the management of urgent and emergent foot and ankle infections. Successful identification of the causative pathogen for all infections is predicated on accurate and appropriate intraoperative specimens.

REFERENCES

1. Patzakis MJ, Wilkins J, Brien WW. Wound site as a predictor of complications following deep nail punctures to the foot. West J Med 1989;150:545–7.
2. Eidelman M, Bialik V, Miller Y, et al. Plantar puncture wounds in children: analysis of 80 hospitalized patients and late sequelae. Isr Med Assoc J 2003;5:268–71.
3. Chang HC, Verhoeven W, Mun CW. Rubber foreign bodies in puncture wounds of the foot in patients wearing rubber-soled shoes. Foot Ankle Int 2001;22:409–14.
4. Armstrong DG, Lavery LA, Quebedeaux TL, et al. Surgical morbidity and the risk of amputation due to infected puncture wounds in diabetic versus nondiabetic adults. J Am Podiatr Med Assoc 1997;87:321–6.
5. Hartemann-Heurtier A, Senneville E. Diabetic foot osteomyelitis. Diabetes Metab 2008;34:87–95.
6. Grayson ML, Gibbons GW, Balogh K, et al. Probing to bone in infected pedal ulcers. A clinical sign of underlying osteomyelitis in diabetic patients. JAMA 1995;273:721–3.
7. Lavery LA, Armstrong DG, Wunderlich RP, et al. Risk factors for foot infections in individuals with diabetes. Diabetes Care 2006;29:1288–93.
8. Gibbons GW. The diabetic foot: amputations and drainage of infection. J Vasc Surg 1987;5:791–3.
9. Citron DM, Goldstein EJC, Merriam CV, et al. Bacteriology of moderate-to-severe diabetic foot infections and in vitro activity of antimicrobial agents. J Clin Microbiol 2007;45:2819–28.
10. Yates C, May K, Hale T, et al. Wound chronicity, inpatient care, and chronic kidney disease predispose to MRSA infection in diabetic foot ulcers. Diabetes Care 2009;32:1907–9.
11. Edmonds M. The treatment of diabetic foot infections: focus on ertapenam. Vasc Health Risk Manag 2009;5:949–63.
12. Dinubile MJ, Lipsky BA. Complicated infections of skin and skin structures: when the infection is more than skin deep. J Antimicrob Chemother 2004;53:ii37–50.
13. Besman AN, Geiger PJ, Canawati H. Prevalence of *Corynebacteria* in diabetic foot infections. Diabetes Care 1992;15:1531–3.
14. Armstrong DG, Lanthier J, Lelievre P, et al. Methicillin-resistant coagulase-negative staphylococcus and its relationship to broad-spectrum oral antibiosis in a predominantly diabetic population. J Foot Ankle Surg 1995;34:353–6.
15. Lipsky BA. Osteomyelitis of the foot in diabetic patients. Clin Infect Dis 1997;25: 1318–26.

16. Nelson SB. Managing diabetic foot infections in an era of increasing microbial resistance. Curr Infect Dis Rep 2009;11:375–82.
17. Dang CN, Prasad YDM, Boulton AJM, et al. Methicillin-resistant *Staphylococcus aureus* in the diabetic foot clinic: a worsening problem. Diabet Med 2003;20: 159–61.
18. Tentolouris N, Petrikkos G, Vallianou N, et al. Prevalance of methicillin-resistant *Staphylococcus aureus* in infected and uninfected diabetic foot ulcers. Clin Microbiol Infect 2006;12:178–96.
19. Stanaway S, Johnson D, Moulik P, et al. Methicillin-resistant *Staphylococcus aureus* (MRSA) isolation from diabetic foot ulcers correlates with nasal MRSA carriage. Diabetes Res Clin Pract 2007;75:47–50.
20. Chang S, Sievert DM, Hageman JC, et al. Infection with vancomycin-resistant *Staphylococcus aureus* containing the vanA resistance gene. N Engl J Med 2003;348:1342–7.
21. Varaiya AY, Dogra JD, Kulkarni MH, et al. Extended-spectrum beta-lactamase-producing *Escherichia coli* and *Klebseilla pneumoniae* in diabetic foot infections. Indian J Pathol Microbiol 2008;51:370–2.
22. Goldner MG. The fate of the second leg in the diabetic amputee. Diabetes 1960; 9:100–3.
23. Whitehouse FW, Jurgensen C, Block MA. The later life of the diabetic amputee. Another look at fate of the second leg. Diabetes 1968;17:520–1.
24. Hasham S, Matteucci P, Stanley PRW, et al. Necrotising fasciitis. BMJ 2005;330: 830–3.
25. Oliver JD. Wound infections caused by *Vibrio vulnificus* and other marine bacteria. Epidemiol Infect 2005;133:383–91.
26. Aragón-Sánchez J, Quintana-Marrero Y, Lázaro-Martínez JL, et al. Necrotizing soft-tissue infections in the feet of patients with diabetes: outcome of surgical treatment and factors associated with limb loss and mortality. Int J Low Extrem Wounds 2009;8:141–6.
27. Armour J, Kersten JR. Diabetic cardiomyopathy and anesthesia. Anesthesiology 2008;108:524–30.
28. Chen D, Lee SL, Peterfreund RA. New therapeutic agents for diabetes mellitus: implications for anesthetic management. Anesth Analg 2009;108:1803–10.

Management of Foot and Ankle Trauma

Zacharia Facaros, DPM[a], John J. Stapleton, DPM[b,c],
Vasilios D. Polyzois, MD, PhD[d], Thomas Zgonis, DPM[e,*]

KEYWORDS

• Trauma management • Foot • Ankle • Surgery • Complications

Foot and ankle trauma remains an area of considerable challenge for the treating physician. The confined soft tissue envelope, coupled with high concentrations of force across small joints, produces injuries associated with substantial long-term morbidity. Trauma is experienced in various facets of daily activities, and each year in the United States, fractures and dislocations account for nearly 1 million hospital admissions.[1] The incidence, severity, and mortality of patients suffering polytrauma injuries have declined significantly in the recent years; however, trauma sustained by the foot did not change in comparable ways.[2] Injuries to the foot and ankle are still commonly underestimated or even unnoticed until late in the acute care setting.

Foot and ankle trauma encompasses a range of injuries that include fractures of 1 or more of the bones that constitute the foot and ankle and damage to muscles, ligaments, tendons, and neurovascular structures. Trauma is routinely detected by the bone and joint defects, but nonosseous injuries can present a complex combination of gross and microscopic pathologic features. Depending on whether the injury resulted from low or high energy or whether it presents as an open (bone protruding through the skin) or a closed fracture, a significant recovery period may be required. A fracture that heals in a deformed position can cause hindrances, including swelling, pain, inability to bear weight, and inability to wear shoes. Surgeons should initiate treatment as soon as possible, which may be the use of various splinting or bracing constructs or even immediate surgical stabilization of the foot and/or ankle in an external fixator, a metal frame that is put in place with pins inserted into the bone.[3] The external fixator preserves proper length of the joint and can be left in place as the treatment of other injuries continues.[3] Edema in the respective extremity must also be controlled, a process that may take up to several weeks. Furthermore, with

---

[a] Division of Podiatric Medicine and Surgery, Department of Orthopaedics, University of Texas Health Science Center at San Antonio, San Antonio, TX, USA
[b] Foot and Ankle Surgery, VSAS Orthopaedics, Allentown, PA, USA
[c] Penn State College of Medicine, Hershey, PA, USA
[d] KAT General Hospital, Athens, Greece
[e] Division of Podiatric Medicine and Surgery, Department of Orthopaedics, University of Texas Health Science Center at San Antonio, San Antonio, TX, USA
* Corresponding author.
E-mail address: zgonis@uthscsa.edu

Perioperative Nursing Clinics 6 (2011) 35–43
doi:10.1016/j.cpen.2010.10.010
1556-7931/11/$ – see front matter © 2011 Elsevier Inc. All rights reserved.

continued developments in surgical techniques pertaining to skeletal fixation by way of anatomically contoured implants, as well as wound care, and vascularized tissue grafts, many lower limbs may now be salvaged with functional results.[4]

This article addresses a few of the cornerstone features pertaining to foot and ankle trauma management: preoperative patient stabilization, operating room (OR) setup, and postoperative care fundamentals.

PREOPERATIVE PATIENT STABILIZATION

Evaluation of a severe injury should entail complete examination of the patient, with assessment and treatment following the Advanced Life Trauma Support System guidelines.[5] Once the patient is systemically under control, the immediate care of a lower extremity injury should include stabilization of the limbs (in anatomic position if possible), along with early reduction of fractures and dislocations. Multidisciplinary teams are contacted to provide valuable input when evaluating severe extremity injuries because of the level of complexity and anatomic system crossover. When applicable, control of active bleeding with direct pressure at the site of hemorrhage and pressure to the more proximal vascular structures should be instituted. Elevation of the injured extremities is generally beneficial but only if the lower extremity is properly immobilized and supported. Expedient restoration of normal circulation along with aggressive systemic resuscitation and stability are the key elements in initial therapy. Medical stabilization should be achieved whenever possible to allow the patient to overcome any initial shock after injury.

Once the patient is admitted to the emergency or fast-track department, the foot and ankle specialist should obtain the complete medical history and perform a thorough physical examination in an expedited fashion if limb salvage is at risk. Host factors such as extreme old and young age, diabetes mellitus, chronic renal failure, obesity, malnutrition, and the use of immunosuppressive medications, such as corticosteroids and chemotherapeutic agents, should be recognized as potentially increasing the risk of infection and can impair overall healing.[6] Ultimately, a meticulous dermatologic, vascular, neurologic, and musculoskeletal evaluation should be performed. After this evaluation, further treatment recommendations and plans are decided, based on a broad classification of the injuries as requiring immediate manipulation or surgical intervention, whether at bedside or in the OR suite; as requiring admittance for close monitoring of stabilization and pain management; or as being able to be securely braced, splinted, or casted and subsequently scheduled for follow-up in the outpatient setting.

In the setting of an acute arterial injury or impending compartment syndrome, elevation is controversial. Compartment syndrome is the compression of nerves, blood vessels, and muscles inside a closed space, leading to tissue death from lack of oxygenation. It may be divided into acute, subacute, and chronic.[7] Classically there are 6 P's associated with compartment syndrome: pain out of proportion to what is expected, paresthesia, pallor, paralysis, pulselessness, and sometimes poikilothermia (failure to thermoregulate).[8] The leg may be divided into 4 compartments, whereas 3 compartments run the entire length of the foot and 5 compartments are confined to the forefoot. The hind foot comprises a single deep calcaneal compartment.[7,9] The average annual incidence of compartment syndrome is 2.3 per 100,000 people.[10] Compartment pressure calculation is the most widely used technique to assist in the diagnosis, measured using the wick catheter technique, with the first clinical symptoms of ischemia appearing at an intracompartmental pressure of 20 to 30 mm Hg more than the patient's diastolic blood pressure.[7,11] Elevation can further decrease arterial flow to the tissue and can theoretically increase pressures and exacerbate the compromised tissue perfusion. Early diagnosis is paramount and calls for a high degree of acuity. Immediate fasciotomy is necessary to provide the patient with the most favorable long-term outcome.

Lacerations can result from a multitude of objects or blunt trauma in which the shear forces on soft tissues can be severe enough to precipitate the degloving injuries. More than 50% of lacerations are caused by blunt injury, and most others by metal, glass, and wood.[12] More than 12 million traumatic wounds are treated annually in the emergency departments throughout the United States.[13] When the laceration is clean, primary repair after thorough debridement is usually possible. However, when significantly torn tissues are involved, wounds may not be amenable for primary closure, especially if a prolonged time has passed or contamination is suspected. Lacerations may involve nerves, tendons, and vascular structures and should be evaluated before repair and then reassessed after surgical approximation. The tetanus status of all patients should be reviewed, and patients should be immunized in accordance with the recommendations of the Centers for Disease Control and Prevention.[14] In addition, ligament and tendon disruption after trauma may result from blunt injury (as seen in sports), lacerations, or mangled extremities.

Fractures and dislocations are common and are solely responsible for almost 1 million hospital admissions each year in the United States.[15] One critical initial decision in managing fractures is determining whether the fracture is open or closed. Open fractures are considered emergencies and require prompt treatment, with surgical debridement and institution of intravenous (IV) antibiotics. The basic principles of treatment of open fractures have held true over the years: immediate wound debridement, early use of antibiotic therapy, skeletal stabilization, and early wound coverage.[16,17] The Gustilo and Anderson classification incorporates the degree of soft tissue loss when evaluating the extent of internal damage, concluding that open fractures require emergency treatment, primary closure may be indicated for type I and II fractures, internal fixation should not be implemented, and antibiotics should be administered before, during, and after surgery.[16]

Unreduced foot and ankle fractures and joint dislocations have the risk of associated soft tissue damage, neurovascular compromise, and limb ischemia. Early reduction and stabilization are essential, with which certain closed fractures can be treated nonoperatively. Severely displaced, malaligned, intra-articular, and unstable fractures are treated surgically to stabilize the deformity, eventually for expedited joint range of motion or ambulation in the postoperative course. These fractures require anatomic reduction to minimize the risk of posttraumatic arthritis.[18]

The greater efficiency in providing emergency rescue to injured patients and the growing safety features of modern cars have significantly reduced the loss of life in high-energy traumas; however, the lower extremity remains susceptible and unprotected. Crush injuries result from significant forces directed at tissues, bursting or shearing the soft tissues, crushing the bones, and causing neurovascular insults. Motor vehicle accidents, falls from a height, and motorcycle accidents are some of the causes of crush injuries.[19,20] Extensive tissue disruption with associated hemorrhage is seen in these cases. Adequate resuscitation and stabilization are essential as a precursor to judgments regarding definitive therapy. Decisions regarding replantation of amputated extremities depend on the specialists' evaluation, and when considering that the lower extremity prostheses function much better than the upper extremity limbs, emphasis is placed on returning the lower extremity to a functional, plantigrade, pain-free limb.[21] Primary amputation is an important consideration in mangled and nonsalvageable extremity injuries. Some criteria for amputation are devitalized muscles and nerves, more than 6 hours of arterial occlusion, or severe associated trauma with persistent hypothermia, acidosis, and coagulopathy, the often referred "life over limb."[4,17,21]

To summarize, trauma to the foot and ankle poses numerous obstacles in determining the most successful outcome for the patient. Because of the long-term effects of these injuries, conscientious diagnosis and treatment should reign supreme, and early diagnosis facilitates proper treatment.

OR SETUP

Proper positioning ensures that the surgical team has ready access to the patient and a clear view of the surgical site. It reduces bleeding, mostly by avoiding venous congestion; minimizes cardiac and respiratory problems; and decreases the risk of pressure-related damage to the skin, nerves, joints, and muscles. Appropriate techniques, used with supportive equipment and devices, contribute to patient safety, according to the Association of Perioperative Registered Nurses.[22] In addition to the type and length of the procedure scheduled and the type of anesthesia to be administered, the patient's age, height, and weight should also be considered. Obese patients have a greater likelihood of nerve and pressure point injuries, whereas the elderly tend to have diminished peripheral circulation, potentially causing further skin compromise.[23,24] The patient's position should provide optimal exposure and access to the operative site, should sustain body alignments and circulatory/respiratory function, and should not compromise neuromuscular structures.

There are 4 basic surgical positions assumed in lower extremity trauma: supine, prone, lateral decubitus, and lateral. Foot and ankle surgeons may also use the Trendelenburg position (patient is supine with head lower than feet) and reverse Trendelenburg position (patient is supine with head higher than feet). Pillows and headrests are pivotal, as is padding to help with hip and leg placement, in which an ipsilateral bump is placed beneath the hip and/or knee for improved access and manipulation. After positioning the patient, final evaluation of body alignment and tissue integrity should be done. The choice of patient positioning is determined by the surgical approach, and the responsibility for overall patient well-being rests with the surgeon, the anesthesiologist, and the nurse who constantly monitors the patient's physiologic status. The circulating nurse may coordinate the details of restraints, support to the extremities, and safe transfers from gurney to bed and vice versa.

Trauma-related surgical procedures require a skilled OR team familiar with the instrumentation involved, which is essential for a safe and expedited pace. Meticulous instrumentation setup is important. Furthermore, choosing the most appropriate operating table is paramount so as to allow unencumbered distal operating field manipulation. The more commonly available table is the Skytron series (Skytron, Grand Rapids, MI, USA) with a variety of accessories available for positioning augmentation.[23,24] A fracture, traction, or radiolucent table may be of use, and each has advantages and disadvantages.[25–27] Various assorted viscoelastic polymer alignment aids may be also required for further assistance.

The OR staff must anticipate the use of intraoperative C-arm fluoroscopy imaging and should ideally be familiar with the associated drapes and positioning aid extensions. The preferred location of the C-arm monitor must be planned accordingly before patient positioning so as to avoid barriers and loss of critical intraoperative moments. Power instrumentation is crucial for most trauma-oriented procedures, and extra batteries and equipment should also be readily available. During the procedure, the surgical team should be reminded not to lean on the patient's trunk or extremities because pressure may further compromise anatomic and physiologic functions. On completion, a 4-person lift or a Davis roller should be used to provide support to the torso, head, and all extremities (**Figs. 1–3**).

POSTOPERATIVE CARE

Soft tissue handling during the perioperative time frame is critical for successful wound closure and healing. Special care should be taken in minimizing soft tissue manipulation. After wound closure, povidone-iodine solution and an absorptive dressing are commonly applied to the wound, followed by a liberal amount of padding involving gauze or cotton material. The foot and ankle are held in a neutral position, and a well-padded short- or long-leg splintor and its cast counterpart may be applied. Compressive Jones-type dressing and elastic wrap, with careful padding along bony prominences, may be used as an alternative.

Edema results from an imbalance in the filtration system between capillary and interstitial spaces, almost always encountered in the postoperative setting. The magnitude of the edema can be related to the severity of the primary trauma and degree of osteosynthesis, if performed.[28] Control of this phenomenon is essential for care of traumatic injuries. Various modalities frequently used for treatment include, but are not limited to, icing and elevation, antiembolic stockings, and pneumatic venous compression pumps.[29–33]

Trauma cases are fairly invasive because of the nature of the injury, often requiring patient admittance to the hospital for proper control of postoperative pain and edema in the acute care setting. IV antibiotics are routinely extended through this period, with strict orders for bed rest and extremity elevation. In addition, this procedure allows for close monitoring of any comorbidities, ensuring that the patient is medically stable and able to rehabilitate before discharge. A period of non–weight bearing is necessary, the course of immobilization routinely extending from 6 to 8 weeks, although a much longer duration is required for more comprehensive reconstruction. Potential complications after foot and ankle trauma may be significant, and more severe injuries may increase the likelihood of various conditions, including, but not limited to, compartment syndrome, posttraumatic arthrosis, avascular necrosis, delayed unions/malunions/nonunions, stiffness, deep venous thrombosis (DVT), persistent pain, and permanent deformity.[17,34]

During the postoperative period, DVT prophylaxis may be administered. One study found that in the postoperative care setting, 44% of surgeons used prophylaxis, most commonly by way of sequential compression devices and low–molecular weight heparin.[35] Risk stratification is instrumental within any perioperative timeline when trauma surgery transpires. Various factors contributing to thrombus predisposition

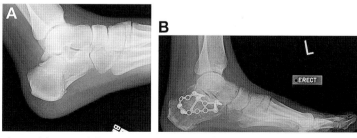

Fig. 1. Calcaneal fracture (*A*) repaired by an open reduction and internal fixation (*B*).

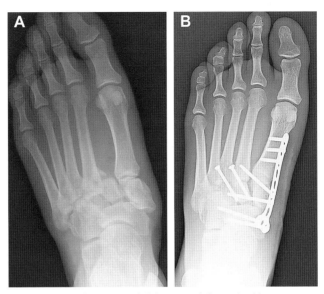

Fig. 2. Tarsometatarsal joint fracture and dislocation (*A*) repaired by an open reduction and internal fixation (*B*).

may be acquired or form from preexisting conditions that solely or together place the patient at risk for a thrombophilic event. Various risk factors associated with venous thromboembolism (VTE) have been well documented, leading to delineation of distinct risk levels.[36] Although little data exist regarding the use of anticoagulant prophylaxis after foot and ankle surgery, it seems to be underused in this subset of surgical patients.

Felcher and colleagues[36] performed a 5-year retrospective analysis of more than 7000 patients undergoing podiatric surgery and found a DVT rate of 3 per 1000

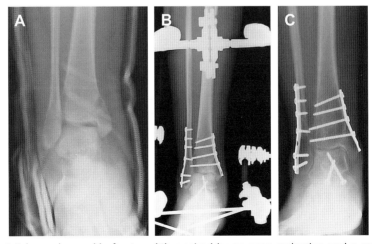

Fig. 3. A talus and an ankle fracture (*A*) repaired by an open reduction and a combined internal and temporary external fixation device (*B, C*).

patients and an overall rate of symptomatic pulmonary embolism (PE) of 0.12%. They concluded that 2 or more risk factors had an overall VTE rate of 1.13% (too low to recommend routine prophylaxis), and if 1 of those risk factors involves prior VTE or if the 2 risk factors are obesity and the use of oral contraceptive pills, then risk increases to approximately 5%, and VTE prophylaxis is recommended.[36] Because thromboembolic events may occur several weeks after surgery, the use of extended prophylaxis postoperatively in the outpatient setting may be beneficial for patients undergoing foot and ankle surgery presenting with additional risk factors for DVT and PE. Mizel and colleagues[37] found that clinically detectable symptoms of thromboembolism occur an average of 34.8 days after surgery (range, 3–70 days).

When supervising trauma-induced surgeries in the postoperative phase, the degree of surgery, severity, healing time, and level of return to activity must be acknowledged. In patients who may have been debilitated for an extended duration, independence and self-determination are central to their restoration of function and return to activities of daily living. Long-term demand of alternative shoe gear and modifications (eg, shock-absorbing soles, arch or cushioned heel supports, or a variety of ankle-foot orthoses and bracing) may be unavoidable. The physical therapy team is instrumental in aiding the rehabilitation of these patients. Restoring joint range of motion and muscle strength is the objective, and emphasis is on neuromuscular coordination and return to normal gait mechanics. A gradual recovery to physical activity that includes function-specific movement is prescribed, with the primary goal of achieving a safe return to motion while minimizing the risk of recurrence or pain.

SUMMARY

Foot and ankle trauma can be devastating to the patient in the perioperative setting and may extend afterward for a long period. As the trauma community increasingly appreciates the incidence of foot and ankle injuries, accurate and timely evaluation of these injuries will assume greater importance in the treatment. The ultimate aim is to restore limb function and get patients back to normal life. To achieve good functional outcomes, it is paramount that the treating team executes proper patient selection, timely reconstruction, and selection of the procedure best suited for the individual.

REFERENCES

1. Brinker MR, O'Connor DP. The incidence of fractures and dislocations referred for orthopaedic services in a capitated population. J Bone Joint Surg Am 2004; 86-A(2):290–7.
2. Tadros AM, Eid HO, Abu-Zidan FM. Epidemiology of foot injury in a high-income developing country. Injury 2010;41(2):137–40.
3. Seibert FJ, Fankhauser F, Elliott B, et al. External fixation in trauma of the foot and ankle. Clin Podiatr Med Surg 2003;20(1):159–80.
4. Ong YS, Levin LS. Lower limb salvage in trauma. Plast Reconstr Surg 2010; 125(2):582–8.
5. American College of Surgeons Committee on Trauma. Abdominal trauma. Advanced Trauma Life Support program. Chicago: American College of Surgeons; 1993. p. 141–55.
6. Cruse PJ, Foord R. A five-year prospective study of 23,649 surgical wounds. Arch Surg 1973;107:206–10.
7. Shadgan B, Menon M, Sanders D, et al. Current thinking about acute compartment syndrome of the lower extremity. Can J Surg 2010;53(5):329–34.

8. Ulmer T. The clinical diagnosis of compartment syndrome of the lower leg: are clinical findings predictive of the disorder? J Orthop Trauma 2002;16(8):572–7.

9. Kamel R, Sakla FB. Anatomical compartments of the sole of the foot. Anat Rec 1961;140:57–64.

10. McQueen MM, Gaston P, Court-Brown CM. Acute compartment syndrome. Who is at risk? J Bone Joint Surg Br 2000;82(2):200–3.

11. Mubarak SJ, Hargens AR, Owen CA, et al. The wick catheter technique for measurement of intramuscular pressure. A new research and clinical tool. J Bone Joint Surg Am 1976;58(7):1016–20.

12. Singer AJ, Hollander JE, Quinn JV. Evaluation and management of traumatic lacerations. N Engl J Med 1997;337(16):1142–8.

13. Stussman BJ. National Hospital Ambulatory Medical Care Survey: 1994 emergency department summary. Advance data from vital and health statistics. No. 275. Hyattsville (MD): National Center for Health Statistics; 1996. DHHS publication (PHS) 96–1250.

14. Centers for Disease Control and Prevention. Diphtheria, tetanus, and pertussis: recommendations for vaccine use and other preventive measures recommendations of the Immunization Practices Advisory Committee. MMWR Morb Mortal Wkly Rep 1991;40(RR–10):1–28.

15. Praemer A, Furner S, Rice DP. Musculoskeletal conditions in the United States. Rosemont (IL): American Academy of Orthopaedic Surgeons; 1999.

16. Gustilo RB, Anderson JT. Prevention of infection in the treatment of one thousand and twenty-five open fractures of long bones: retrospective and prospective analyses. J Bone Joint Surg Am 1976;58:453–8.

17. Yaremchuk MJ, Brumback RJ, Manson PN, et al. Acute and definitive management of traumatic osteocutaneous defects of the lower extremity. Plast Reconstr Surg 1987;80(1):1–14.

18. Makwana NK, Bhowal B, Harper WM, et al. Conservative versus operative treatment for displaced ankle fractures in patients over 55 years of age. A prospective, randomised study. J Bone Joint Surg Br 2001;83:525–9.

19. Wilson LS Jr, Mizel MS, Michelson JD. Foot and ankle injuries in motor vehicle accidents. Foot Ankle Int 2001;22(8):649–52.

20. Ferreira RC, Sakata MA, Costa MT, et al. Long-term results of salvage surgery in severely injured feet. Foot Ankle Int 2010;31(2):113–23.

21. Gregory RT, Gould RJ, Peclet M, et al. The mangled extremity syndrome (M.E.S.): a severity grading system for multisystem injury of the extremity. J Trauma 1985; 25(12):1147–50.

22. Association of Operating Room Nurses. Recommended practices for positioning the patient in the perioperative practice setting. 2005 Standards, recommended practices, and guidelines. Denver (CO): AORN Inc; 2005. p. 427–32.

23. Dybec RB. Intraoperative positioning and care of the obese patient. Plast Surg Nurs 2004;24(3):118–22.

24. Frey C, Zamora J. The effects of obesity on orthopaedic foot and ankle pathology. Foot Ankle Int 2007;28(9):996–9.

25. Blasier RD, Ramsey JR, White RR. Comparison of radiolucent and fracture tables in the treatment of slipped capital femoral epiphysis. J Pediatr Orthop 2004;24(6): 642–4.

26. Nichter L, Bindiger A, Morgan R. Nonorthopedic use of the fracture table. Ann Plast Surg 1992;29(4):376–7.

27. Servant C. How not to be stumped by the traction table. Ann R Coll Surg Engl 2005;87(2):142.

28. Szczesny G, Olszewski WL, Deszczyński J. [Post-traumatic lymphatic and venous drainage changes in persistent edema of lower extremities]. Chir Narzadow Ruchu Ortop Pol 2000;65(3):315–25 [in Polish].
29. Gardner AM, Fox RH, Lawrence C, et al. Reduction of post-traumatic swelling and compartment pressure by impulse compression of the foot. J Bone Joint Surg Br 1990;72(5):810–5.
30. Stöckle U, Hoffmann R, Raschke M, et al. [Intermittent impulse compression. An alternative in therapy of post-traumatic and postoperative edema]. Chirurg 1996; 67(5):539–45 [in German].
31. Kazmi SS, Stranden E, Kroese AJ, et al. Edema in the lower limb of patients operated on for proximal femoral fractures. J Trauma 2007;62(3):701–7.
32. Mayrovitz HN, Macdonald JM. Medical compression: effects on pulsatile leg blood flow. Int Angiol 2010;29(5):436–41.
33. Saedon M, Stansby G. Post-thrombotic syndrome: prevention is better than cure. Phlebology 2010;25(Suppl 1):14–9.
34. Soohoo NF, Farng E, Zingmond DS. Incidence of pulmonary embolism following surgical treatment of metatarsal fractures. Foot Ankle Int 2010;31(7):600–3.
35. Wolf JM, DiGiovanni CW. A survey of orthopedic surgeons regarding DVT prophylaxis in foot and ankle trauma surgery. Orthopedics 2004;27(5):504–8.
36. Felcher AH, Mularski RA, Mosen DM, et al. Incidence and risk factors for venous thromboembolic disease in podiatric surgery. Chest 2009;135:917–22.
37. Mizel MS, Temple HT, Micheison JD, et al. Thromboembolism after foot and ankle surgery. Clin Orthop 1998;348:180–5.

Plastic Surgical Techniques for the Foot and Ankle

John J. Stapleton, DPM[a,b,*], Crystal L. Ramanujam, DPM[c]

KEYWORDS

- Plastic reconstruction • Foot • Ankle • Surgery
- Advancement flaps • Diabetic ulcer

ADVANCED PLASTIC SURGICAL TECHNIQUES: INDICATIONS AND CONTRAINDICATIONS

Random advancement or rotational flaps, split-thickness skin grafts, and local muscle and pedicle flaps are commonly used for closing a complicated foot and ankle wound. Local flaps are typically based on the geometric designs, the mobility and condition of the surrounding soft tissues, the nature of their movement, and the angiosomes of the foot.[1,2] Local flaps can be advanced, transposed, or rotated to provide soft tissue coverage of the defect.

Split-thickness skin grafts can be used in wounds with exposed granulation tissue, dermis, fascia, muscle, peritenon, paratenon, and periosteum. A split-thickness skin graft may not be used in wounds with greater than 5 mm of exposed bone or tendon, over adipose tissue, and over weight-bearing areas. The main prerequisites for split-thickness skin grafting are the presence of a granular wound bed with no drainage, malodor, periwound erythema, edema, and no systemic signs of infection.[3] Granulation tissue is an indicator of skin graft readiness and survival. Granulation tissue is absent if the wound bed is not well perfused or if infection remains.

The pedicle flap is used predominately for durable soft tissue closure of the weight-bearing aspect of the foot and is useful when performed in conjunction with a skeletal reconstruction of the midfoot[4,5] and for closure of calcaneal defects.[6] The main advantage of a pedicle flap is that extensive soft tissue coverage to the plantar aspect of the foot can be provided without the microvascular anastomosis that is required of a free tissue transfer (**Fig. 1**).

Absolute contraindications to surgical wound closure via plastic surgical techniques include vascular insufficiency despite endovascular or vascular surgery, complicated

[a] Foot and Ankle Surgery, VSAS Orthopaedics, Allentown, PA, USA
[b] Penn State College of Medicine, Hershey, PA, USA
[c] Division of Podiatric Medicine and Surgery, Department of Orthopaedics, University of Texas Health Science Center at San Antonio, San Antonio, TX, USA
* Corresponding author. Foot and Ankle Surgery, VSAS Orthopaedics, Allentown, PA.
E-mail address: Jostaple@hotmail.com

Perioperative Nursing Clinics 6 (2011) 45–49
doi:10.1016/j.cpen.2010.10.008 **periopnursing.theclinics.com**
1556-7931/11/$ – see front matter © 2011 Published by Elsevier Inc.

A
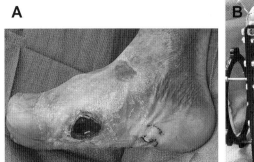

B
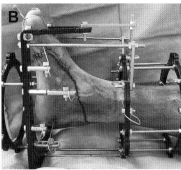

Fig. 1. A plantar midfoot soft tissue defect associated with a Charcot deformity and instability of the tarsometatarsal joint developed after an imbalanced forefoot amputation (*A*). The residual foot required both soft tissue and osseous reconstruction for limb salvage. The patient underwent initial ulcer excision with intraoperative bone biopsy and deep soft tissue and bone cultures. A staged tarsometatarsal arthrodesis and reconstruction with local random flap was performed. Circular external fixation was used for osseous stabilization and to adequately off-load the soft tissues, permitting close observation in the postoperative period (*B*).

cardiac issues, nonambulatory patients, unsalvageable feet, and noncompliant patients.

PERIOPERATIVE CONSIDERATIONS

The overall management of most foot and ankle wounds is best handled by a multidisciplinary team, which may include foot and ankle specialists, vascular surgeons, plastic surgeons, trauma surgeons, burn specialists, internists, nephrologists, endocrinologists, cardiologists, physiatrists, wound-care nurses, physical therapists, psychologists, and nutritionists. Comorbidities must be managed as a team, and the patient optimized to ensure successful wound healing.

The circulating nurse assesses the patient and verifies the patient's identity and accompanying history. It is important to understand the role of each team member and the multifactorial management that is typically rendered to manage a foot and ankle wound. For example, a patient who recently had a lower extremity arterial bypass to treat arterial insufficiency may present for a wound debridement and closure. In normal circumstances, a tourniquet may be used; however, the nursing staff should determine if a tourniquet may be used in this case because it may compromise the lower extremity bypass. The conclusion is that multiple services are typically treating and managing these patients, and the nurse assessment needs to organize the rendered treatment among the surgical team when preparing the patient for the operating theater. A comprehensive nursing care plan can be established once a detailed history and physical examination has been obtained and documented from the medical chart.

The circulating nurse confirms the proposed procedure, and the surgeon should verify the procedure and mark the surgical lower extremity. At that point, all questions of the family and the patient should be addressed. The circulating nurse notes the results of any abnormal laboratory studies. In particular, if the hemoglobin and hematocrit levels of the patient are decreased, it is discussed with the surgeon and anesthesiologist to confirm that the blood typing and cross-matching for packed red blood cells are also available at the time of surgery. The need for and the most appropriate antibiotic for prophylaxis should be determined, and the antibiotic should be administered in a timely manner. Over-the-counter medications used by the patient, medical or food allergies, previous surgical complications, and social history are also documented.

OPERATIVE SETTING AND PREPARATION

The circulating nurse, along with the scrub technician, prepares the sterile surgical field. The nursing team is informed of the instrumentation in advance so that it is prepared and readily available during the procedure. Equipment needs can vary greatly depending on the adjunctive procedures that may need to be performed. For cases that require soft tissue and bone debridements, basic orthopedic trays that include osteotomes, rongeurs, and curettes are sufficient. For bone resections and/or arthrodesis, sagittal and/or oscillating saws are typically used, with the size and shape of the blade determined in advance. In addition, internal and/or external fixation for osseous stability may be used and must be arranged in advance by the surgeon. At present, external fixation is used more often for lower extremity wounds to provide adequate off-loading of the soft tissues and facilitate close observation and postoperative wound care. It is advantageous to arrange a separate table for instrumentation and equipment that are typically required for external fixation cases because the trays encompass a large surface area. For more complicated wound closure techniques, such as reconstruction with random local and pedicle flaps, a basic plastic surgery and/or neurosurgery tray should be available. Cases that require a split-thickness skin graft need a power dermatome with an appropriately sized blade and a mesher. A high-pressure pulse lavage system or cystoscopy tubing is used for adequate irrigation and assembled on the surgical field along with the required amount of saline, which is hung from an intravenous pole. An antibiotic added to the solution has not been shown to be advantageous but still remains as the surgeon's preference regarding its use.[7] A large basin and a radiograph cassette cover should also be used along with suction to prevent the aerosolization of bacteria particles during irrigation via a pulse lavage. It is beneficial to use a Mayo stand or an additional table along with the traditional sterile table, which allows an area to remain sterile after surgical debridement and pulse lavage irrigation. This technique prevents contamination from the equipment used for wound closure that was previously used to surgically excise tissue or bone that may have had high bacterial counts. Culture swabs and specimen cups should be available when anticipating the collection of soft tissue or bone cultures and tissue specimens for histopathologic examination.

Electrocautery should be established for each patient. Often, diabetic patients with foot complications are also cardiac patients with pacemakers. The use of a magnet and/or bipolar cautery may be warranted in these select cases and should be discussed with the surgeon and the anesthesiologist to prevent cardiac complications. The anesthesia care provider and the circulating nurse typically provide the transport of the patient to the operating room when ready. The patient is typically positioned supine unless the soft tissue coverage involves the heel region or the posterior lower leg, in which case a prone position or lateral decubital position is needed.

After patient positioning, a pneumatic sequential compression device (SCD) is used on the nonsurgical lower extremity to further prevent the incidence of deep vein thrombosis (DVT) and pulmonary embolism (PE) in the postoperative period. Although the published rates of DVT and PE after foot and ankle surgery are relatively low, many patients with these conditions may have significant risk factors that can increase the chance of these events; therefore, mechanical and pharmacologic therapy may be indicated.[8] Contraindications for an SCD are severe arterial insufficiency, recent lower extremity bypass or endovascular procedure, and trauma to the affected leg. A thigh tourniquet is used for patients who are under general anesthesia or have received a spinal anesthetic. An ankle or calf tourniquet is placed if an ankle block is to be performed. It is important to apply tourniquets far proximal from the operative field site and keep tourniquet inflation times as short as possible to decrease risk of complications such as neuropraxia, edema, and vascular injury.[9] Tourniquets are usually inflated after the initial surgical debridement, irrigation, and procurement of the intraoperative cultures. The tourniquet is deflated after meticulous flap dissection to further assess the viability of the flap and provide adequate hemostasis before closure.[10] Topical thrombin and gel foam should be readily available if needed for additional hemostasis. Appropriate sterile preparation of the surgical lower extremity is performed by the circulating nurse. The type of solution used is usually based on the surgeon's preference because studies have shown mixed results regarding efficacy.[11,12]

It is paramount for the surgeon and the circulating nurse to discuss the specifics of surgical instrumentation that is needed, suture supplies, and/or use of intraoperative imaging before the surgery is initiated. Also, postoperative dressings and splinting materials should be available and ready in the room to further prevent prolonged operating time and anesthesia recovery. An operating room that is set up with the necessary basic instrumentation greatly facilitates surgery in these high-risk patients.

POSTOPERATIVE CARE

The patient's vital signs, laboratory studies, culture and sensitivity results, and daily clinical status are documented. It is advantageous to have the patient first evaluated by the nursing staff. The nursing care provider is trained to observe and relay to the physician the patient's demeanor, mood, and obvious problems. The surgical team can then enter the room better prepared to interact with the patient. Emphasis on the patient's dressing changes, wound care, physical therapy, limb position, shower privileges, and sampling for laboratory tests are discussed at the bedside. A multidisciplinary approach continues throughout the postoperative period to ensure a successful outcome. A protocol with guidelines is established by all team members so that a mutual understanding is established regarding the postoperative care. Patients need ongoing support and validation throughout the recovery period to ensure a functional recovery and prevent related complications.

Discharge from the hospital should represent an accomplishment for the patient. It should include a prognosis for the patient along with a discussion of the remaining postoperative course. The patient should be given instructions for follow-up and daily or weekly monitoring of the surgical procedure, medications, ancillary services, ambulatory status, work and social restrictions, and bathing instructions. The patient should also be given instructions on identifying signs of infection and ways of contacting the surgical team if problems arise.

SUMMARY

Many surgical options exist for the closure of soft tissue defects of the foot and ankle. It is important to understand the multiple factors in procedure selection and throughout the perioperative period. The integration of all team members enables them to be well informed and prepared to ensure a successful outcome.

REFERENCES

1. Attinger CE, Evans KK, Bulan E, et al. Angiosomes of the foot and ankle and clinical implications for limb salvage: reconstruction, incisions, and revascularization. Plast Reconstr Surg 2006;117(Suppl 7):261–93.
2. Capobianco CM, Ramanujam CL, Zgonis T. A simple adjunct to a plantar local random flap for submetatarsal ulcers. Clin Podiatr Med Surg 2010;27:167–72.
3. Ramanujam CL, Stapleton JJ, Kilpadi KL, et al. Split-thickness skin grafts for closure of diabetic foot and ankle wounds: a retrospective review of 83 patients. Foot Ankle Spec 2010;3(5):231–40.
4. Banerjee R, Waterman B, Nelson J. Reconstruction of massive midfoot bone and soft tissue loss as a result of blast injury. J Foot Ankle Surg 2010;49:301–4.
5. Zgonis T, Roukis TS, Stapleton JJ, et al. Combined lateral column arthrodesis, medial plantar artery flap, and circular external fixation for Charcot midfoot collapse with chronic plantar ulceration. Adv Skin Wound Care 2008;21:521–5.
6. Skef Z, Ecker HA Jr, Graham WP 3rd. Heel coverage by a plantar myocutaneous island pedicle flap. J Trauma 1983;23:466–72.
7. Owens BD, White DW, Wenke JC. Comparison of irrigation solutions and devices in a contaminated musculoskeletal wound survival model. J Bone Joint Surg Am 2009;91:92–8.
8. Slaybaugh RS, Beasley BD, Massa EG. Deep venous thrombosis risk assessment, incidence, and prophylaxis in foot and ankle surgery. Clin Podiatr Med Surg 2003;20:269–89.
9. Smith TO, Hing CB. The efficacy of the tourniquet in foot and ankle surgery? A systematic review and meta-analysis. Foot Ankle Surg 2010;16:3–8.
10. Zgonis T, Stapleton JJ, Rodriguez RH, et al. Plastic surgery reconstruction of the diabetic foot. AORN J 2008;87:951–66.
11. Ostrander RV, Botte MJ, Brage ME. Efficacy of surgical preparation solutions in foot and ankle surgery. J Bone Joint Surg Am 2005;87:980–5.
12. Ostrander RV, Brage ME, Botte MJ. Bacterial skin contamination after surgical preparation in foot and ankle surgery. Clin Orthop Relat Res 2003;406:246–52.

Orthobiologics in Foot and Ankle Surgery

Claire M. Capobianco, DPM[a],*, Thomas Zgonis, DPM[b,c]

KEYWORDS

• Orthobiologics • Nonunion • Diabetes • Foot • Ankle • Surgery

A discussion of the major advances in the realm of foot and ankle surgery in the last 2 decades would likely include intramedullary (IM) fixation, widespread use of Ilizarov external fixation, improved implants, and orthobiologics. All these broad categories have improved surgeons' management of challenging pathologic conditions, and many have spawned the development of an entire industry. More recently, external fixation, IM fixation, and locking plate technology have conferred even further stability across fracture or fusion sites and have aided in minimizing deleterious micromotion. Despite years of advances in fixation, the insatiable quest for improved outcomes has fueled the development of an entirely new approach, one that encompasses the addition of living matrices, cells, and proteins in an attempt to improve wound healing and bony fusions. This new frontier is the rapidly expanding realm of orthobiologics.

Orthobiologics are also referred to in the literature as bioadjuvants, bioengineered tissue alternatives, and living tissue substitutes.[1] Broadly, orthobiologic products use living cells or subcomponents of living tissue or fluids and are thought to enhance healing in native tissues. The products can be arbitrarily categorized into those that are used in bone healing and those that are used for wound or soft tissue repair. This article reviews the most common categories, applications, and advantages and disadvantages of these products.

BONE HEALING

A cursory understanding of basic osseous repair is integral to an understanding of the orthobiologic products available. Osteoinduction, osteogenesis, and osteoconduction

[a] Orthopaedic Associates of Southern Delaware, 17005 Old Orchard Road, Lewes, DE 19958, USA
[b] Division of Podiatric Medicine and Surgery, Department of Orthopaedics, University of Texas Health Science Center at San Antonio, 7703 Floyd Curl Drive, MSC 7776, San Antonio, TX 78829, USA
[c] Research and Reconstructive Foot and Ankle Fellowships, University of Texas Health Science Center at San Antonio, 7703 Floyd Curl Drive, MSC 7776, San Antonio, TX 78829, USA
* Corresponding author.
E-mail address: coatescm@gmail.com

Perioperative Nursing Clinics 6 (2011) 51–57
doi:10.1016/j.cpen.2010.10.007
1556-7931/11/$ – see front matter © 2011 Elsevier Inc. All rights reserved.

are the 3 properties by which any type of graft (autogeneic or allogeneic) can affect bony healing. Osteoinduction is the ability to convert mesenchymal precursor cells to bone-producing osteoblasts. Osteogenesis is the ability to form bone de novo from cells within the graft, and osteoconduction is the ability of a product to act as a conduit for bone-forming cells. Some products contain one or more of these properties, whereas others focus on providing relatively more of a certain property.

Autogenous products include bone marrow aspirate, cortical or cancellous autograft, and osteochondral plugs. In foot and ankle surgery, autograft is easily harvested from the distal tibia, from posterior calcaneus, and/or locally at the sites of arthrodesis preparation. However, the rich pluripotential cells found in the marrow of long bones elsewhere in the body is developmentally scant in bones of the distal lower extremity and foot. As such, the relative concentrations of the osteoinductive and osteogenic growth factors and signaling cells can be questioned, even though osteoblasts are not scarce. Conversely, bone marrow aspirate, typically obtained from the iliac crest, is rich in osteoinductive and osteogenic qualities but lacks structure and conductivity. The applications of different types of autogenous bone grafts depends on the primary characteristics desired for the graft; for example, corticocancellous calcaneal or iliac crest graft offers significant structural and volumetric support, whereas cancellous distal tibial graft is better suited for in situ arthrodeses.

Autogeneic osteochondral plugs are frequently obtained from the ipsilateral knee or plantarmedial aspect of the nonarticular portion of the talar head and are used for repair of osteochondral defects, usually in the talar dome or first metatarsal head. These plugs are osteoinductive, osteogeneic, and osteoconductive. Allogeneic osteochondral plugs are also widely available from tissue banks and offer the surgeon largely the same advantages, excepting osteoinductive capability, but with less patient morbidity.

Allogeneic grafts are available in multiple preparations, including fresh, frozen or freshly frozen, demineralized, or lyophilized forms. In foot and ankle surgery, the most frequent structural corticocancellous grafts used include talus, iliac crest, calcaneus, and femoral head grafts. Preparation of the graft affects its qualities. Fresh grafts are osteoinductive, osteogeneic, and osteoconductive. Freshly frozen grafts may lack inductive qualities, depending on the exact method of graft preparation. Allogeneic grafts, such as talus, iliac crest, and femoral head grafts, are preferred by some for complex revisional rearfoot surgeries (**Fig. 1**).

Allogeneic demineralized grafts are acellular and particulate and contain demineralized bone matrix (DBM), bone morphogenetic proteins (BMPs), growth factors, collagens, and proteoglycans. BMPs are classified under the transforming growth factor β category, and multiple BMPs have been shown to aggressively promote de novo bone formation via their beneficial effects on stem cell precursors.[2] The presence of DBM, BMPs, and growth factors in demineralized grafts adds osteoinductive capacity to nonstructural osteoconductivity and, when indicated, these grafts are often used in combination with a structural type graft.[3,4]

Because large quantities of BMPs are necessary for the desired effects, the isolation and concentration of specific BMPs has spurred further industrial development. The formulation of a product consisting solely of the osteoinductive BMPs is understood to improve initiation of stem cell differentiation.[3] The use of BMPs in spinal fusion, in open fractures in long and craniofacial bones, and in long and scaphoid bone nonunions has been well described.[5,6] There is scant literature defining the appropriate indications for the use of expensive BMP isolates in the foot and ankle, but early studies have described successful application in patients considered at high risk for foot and ankle nonunions.[2] In addition, a role for BMP-7 in cartilage repair in the lower extremity has been proposed, and early in vitro and animal research seems promising.[7]

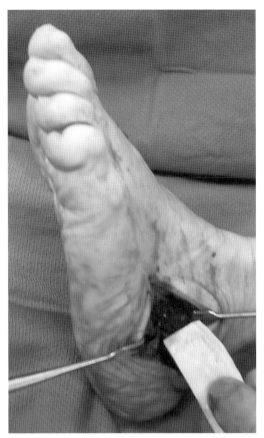

Fig. 1. An intraoperative picture showing an allogeneic tricortical ilac crest for rearfoot reconstruction.

Allogeneic lyophilized grafts are also devoid of any viable cells but lack growth factors and DBM and thus, are solely osteoconductive. The use of lyophilized grafts is common to arthrodeses throughout the foot and ankle. Allografts of any type offer the obvious benefit of decreased surgical morbidity to the patient, and improvements in the screening, irradiation, and treatment of the grafts has diminished the risk of disease transmission to less than one in a million.[4]

Platelets have also been targeted as adjuncts for bone healing, especially in combination with DBM. Platelets release multiple growth factors from alpha granules including, but not limited to, platelet-derived growth factor (PDGF), epidermal growth factor, insulinlike growth factor 1, granulocyte colony stimulating factor, and vascular endothelial growth factor.[8] These growth factors are thought to act on bone via cellular chemotactic interactions and to enhance cellular signaling, angiogenesis, matrix production, and substrate remodeling.[3,8] As such, the application of a concentrated form of autogenous platelet-rich plasma (PRP) in addition to concentrated osteoinductive BMPs is attractive (**Fig. 2**).

Synthetic calcium salt matrices offer osteoconductive scaffold properties for the new bone but lack any inductive or de novo bone-forming ability. Although not technically biologic, these types of products are still used when structural conduits are

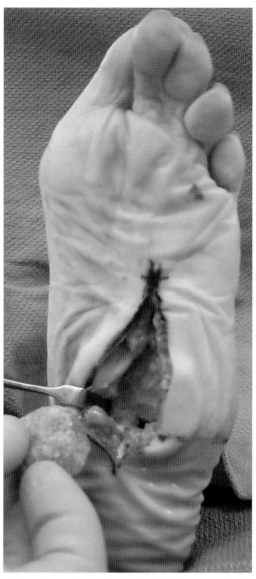

Fig. 2. An intraoperative picture of an allogeneic DBM bone graft mixed with an autogenous PRP for a Charcot foot reconstruction.

needed, and are more frequently being used in combination with PRP, DBM, or BMP. The major benefits of synthetic grafts include availability, storage, and absence of potential disease transmission. This type of graft may also be impregnated with antibiotics when needed. Depending on the specific formulation calcium sulfate, calcium phosphate, and composite products may integrate with native tissues, even though the formation of draining sinuses and graft frailty is well reported.[4] Xenografts of bovine or equine origin are also available and offer primarily osteoconductive qualities, but these are not widely used at present.[4]

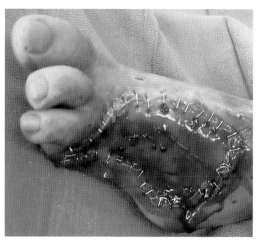

Fig. 3. An intraoperative picture showing a collagen-glycosaminoglycan biodegradable matrix for soft tissue reconstruction of the diabetic foot.

WOUND AND SOFT TISSUE HEALING

The bioengineered tissues used in wound healing are all composed of types of micro-scaffolds to encourage depth reduction and epibolization of the wound bed (**Fig. 3**). Some of the products contain living human cells such as fibroblasts and keratinocytes and can be engineered in mono or bilayer formulations to mimic the native dermis and epidermis. The most common of these products include Apligraf (Organogenesis Inc, Canton, MA, USA), Dermagraft (Advanced BioHealing Inc, La Jolla, CA, USA), Epicel (Genzyme Tissue Repair Corp, Cambridge, MA, USA), and OrCel (Ortec International Inc, New York, NY, USA).[1,9] The most extensively studied of these products have earned the Food and Drug Administration's approval for use in diabetic foot ulcerations and chronic venous stasis wounds.[1,9,10] Other tissues are acellular in nature but contain allogeneic (GraftJacket [Wright Medical Technology Inc Arlington, TX, USA]) or xenogeneic (Integra [Integra Life Sciences Inc, Plainsboro, NJ, USA], OrthA-DAPT [Pegasus Biologics Inc, Irvine, CA, USA], EZ-Derm [Brennen Medical Inc, St Paul, MN, USA]) collagen scaffolds, skin (Alloderm [LifeCell Corp/Kinetic Concepts Inc, Woodlands, TX, USA]), submucosa (Oasis [HEALTHPOINT Ltd, Fort Worth, TX, USA]), or peptides (Biobrane [Dow Hickam/Bertek Pharmaceuticals, Sugar Land, TX, USA]).[1,9] Some of the products tout the presence of active growth factors to aid wound and soft tissue healing.[1,10] In addition to wounds, the more durable products have also been successfully used as adjuncts in musculotendinous repair surgery in the lower extremity.

In the foot and ankle, the acellular products are typically applied to deeper, higher-volume, more complex, or recalcitrant wounds, and the cellular products tend to be more suitable for superficial wounds.[11] The bioengineered tissues are all costly; thorough understanding of appropriate wound preparation and staging is essential for judicious use of these technologies. Also, most wound care matrices normally appear like slough or coagulum after application, and this knowledge is crucial to avoid inadvertent debridement of the desired tissue.

Similarly, the growth factors previously described in PRP are also understood to be efficacious in wound and soft tissue healing.[8] As such, activated PRP has been reported to be applied directly on wound surfaces before application of bioengineered tissues[1,12] or skin grafts.[13] Isolated growth factors, such as recombinant human PGDF, (marketed commercially in gel form as bercaplermin [Regranex; Systagenix, Quincy, MA, USA]) have been used successfully both as first-line and secondary treatment of diabetic foot ulcers and have been found to be cost-effective and efficacious when compared with traditional wound care.[14]

Other orthobiologics focus on lessening the negative effects of bioactive compounds in chronic wounds. Matrix metalloproteases (MMPs) are a complicated superfamily of enzymes that are active in all phases of wound healing.[15,16] The excessive proteolytic activity of certain MMPs is postulated to result in detrimental degradation of extracellular matrix and senescence of chronic wounds.[15] For this reason, therapies directed at the inhibition of MMPs, including stimulation of native protease inhibitors and topically applied protease inhibitors (PROMOGRAN PRISMA, [Ethicon Inc, Cornelia, GA, USA]), have become commonplace in wound care management.

NEW HORIZONS

The field of orthobiologics is constantly growing. In small studies involving the knee, developments in matrix-induced autologous chondrocyte implantation grafts have shown promising midterm and long-term outcomes.[17] In diabetic rats, the application of specific concentrated recombinant PDGF isolates is showing encouraging effects on fracture healing.[18] Concentrated bench research into the isolation of autogenous osteoprogenitor cells is also ongoing, as is work with collagen and stem cell formulations for tendon and ligament repair.[19] An impressive case report detailing the initial success in whole bone tissue engineering of a distal hallux phalanx from harvested distal radius periosteal progenitor cells has already been published.[19,20] In addition, the use of allogeneic, irradiated, leukocyte-depleted, ABO- and RhD-matched, human thrombin–activated PRP has been successfully described and is advantageous in the larger quantities available for use during surgery.[8]

SUMMARY

A vast spectrum of orthobiologic products exists to enhance bone and soft tissue healing. Reported outcomes have suggested that these adjuncts may be beneficial in challenging pathologic conditions, revisional surgeries, or in patients at high risk for complications after bone or wound repair surgery in the foot and ankle. More research is needed to better delineate the indications and efficacy of the newer products, with special regard to combinations of products. The continued expansion of the orthobiologic realm is expected to commensurate with cellular and subcellular academic dissection of difficult pathologic conditions.

REFERENCES

1. Steinberg JS, Werber B, Kim PJ. Bioengineered alternative tissues for surgical management of diabetic foot ulceration. In: Zgonis T, editor. Surgical reconstruction of the diabetic foot and ankle. Philadelphia: Lippincott, Williams & Wilkins; 2009. p. 105–9.
2. Schuberth JM, DiDomenico LA, Mendicino RW. The utility and effectiveness of bone morphogenetic protein in foot and ankle surgery. J Foot Ankle Surg 2009; 48:309–14.
3. Han B, Woodell-May J, Ponticello M, et al. The effect of thrombin activation of platelet-rich plasma on demineralized bone matrix osteoinductivity. J Bone Joint Surg Am 2009;91:1459–70.

4. Cook EA, Cook JJ. Bone graft substitutes and allografts for reconstruction of the foot and ankle. Clin Podiatr Med Surg 2009;26:589–605.
5. White AP, Hall JA, Whang PG, et al. Clinical applications of BMP-7/OP-1 in fractures, nonunions and spinal fusion. Int Orthop 2007;31:735–41.
6. Bishop GB, Einhorn TA. Current and future clinical applications of bone morphogenetic proteins in orthopaedic trauma surgery. Int Orthop 2007;31:721–7.
7. Chubinskaya S, Hurtig M, Rueger DC. OP-1/BMP-7 in cartilage repair. Int Orthop 2007;31:773–81.
8. Rožman P, Bolta Z. Use of platelet growth factors in treating wounds and soft tissue injuries. Acta Dermatovenerol Alp Panonica Adriat 2007;16:156–65.
9. Lee KH. Tissue-engineered human living skin substitutes: development and clinical application. Yonsei Med J 2000;41:774–9.
10. Zaulyanov L, Kirsner RS. A review of a bi-layered living cell treatment (Apligraf®) in the treatment of venous leg ulcers and diabetic foot ulcers. Clin Interv Aging 2007;2:93–8.
11. Capobianco CM, Stapleton JJ, Zgonis T. Soft tissue reconstruction pyramid in the diabetic foot. Foot Ankle Spec 2010;3(5):241–8.
12. Lacci KM, Dardik A. Platelet-rich plasma: support for its use in wound healing. Yale J Biol Med 2010;83:1–9.
13. Schade VL, Roukis TS. Use of platelet-rich plasma with split-thickness skin grafts in the high-risk patient. Foot Ankle Spec 2008;1:155–9.
14. Lantis JC 2nd, Boone D, Gendics C, et al. Analysis of patient cost for recombinant human platelet-derived growth factor therapy as the first-line treatment of the insured patient with a diabetic foot ulcer. Adv Skin Wound Care 2009;22:167–71.
15. Harding KG, Morris HL, Patel GK. Healing chronic wounds. BMJ 2002;324:160–3.
16. Gill SE, Parks WC. Metalloproteinases and their inhibitors: regulators of wound healing. Int J Biochem Cell Biol 2008;40:1334–47.
17. Genovese E, Ronga M, Angeretti MG, et al. Matrix-induced autologous chondrocyte implantation of the knee: mid-term and long-term follow-up by MR arthrography. Skeletal Radiol 2010. [Epub ahead of print].
18. Al-Zube L, Breitbart EA, O'Connor JP, et al. Recombinant human platelet-derived growth factor BB (rhPDGF-BB) and beta-tricalcium phosphate/collagen matrix enhance fracture healing in a diabetic rat model. J Orthop Res 2009;27:1074–81.
19. Vacanti CA, Bonassar LJ, Vacanti MP, et al. Replacement of an avulsed phalanx with tissue-engineered bone. N Engl J Med 2001;344:1511–4.
20. Oakes BW. Orthopedic tissue engineering: from laboratory to clinic. MJA 2004;180:S35–8.

Perioperative Considerations for External Fixation in Foot and Ankle Surgery

Claire M. Capobianco, DPM[a],*, Zacharia Facaros, DPM[b],
Thomas Zgonis, DPM[b]

KEYWORDS

• External fixation • Foot • Ankle • Diabetes • Plastic surgery

HISTORY

Circular external fixation, first described by Dr Gavril Ilizarov in the 1950s, incorporates the temporary use of externally tensioned transosseous pins or wires to control bone segments. Circular rings and bars are secured to these wires outside the body in often-complicated constructs for stabilization or directed motion.[1] The applications for external fixation in the foot and ankle are wide ranging and include acute fracture immobilization, soft tissue immobilization, angular correction of congenital deformity, arthrodesis, revisional surgery, and reconstructive surgery in high-risk patients.

Ilizarov originally experimented with external fixation in tibial osteotomies in dogs and with successes, advanced to treating complex multisegmental limb deformities in humans. More than anyone else's experiments of that era, his experiments aided in defining the characteristics of bone as a living tissue, especially in response to stress and strain.[2,3] Importantly, he described the novel process of bone transport with external fixation, which allowed him to then experiment with surgical uses for novel bone formation. Decades later, his discoveries and thought processes have revolutionized surgical approaches to congenital deformities; trauma; and complicated deformities in the upper extremity, lower extremity, and spine.

[a] Orthopaedic Associates of Southern Delaware, 17005 Old Orchard Road, Lewes, DE, USA
[b] Division of Podiatric Medicine and Surgery, Department of Orthopaedics, University of Texas Health Science Center at San Antonio, San Antonio, TX, USA
* Corresponding author.
E-mail address: coatescm@gmail.com

Perioperative Nursing Clinics 6 (2011) 59–66
doi:10.1016/j.cpen.2010.10.006
1556-7931/11/$ – see front matter © 2011 Elsevier Inc. All rights reserved.

ADVANTAGES/DISADVANTAGES

External fixation is a major tool in the foot and ankle surgeon's approach to many varied pathologies. The interchangeable multisegmental nature of external fixators allows for adaptability and creativity on the part of the surgeon to best address the components of the deformity. External fixators can be designed to allow for acute or gradual motion to correct osseous or soft tissue deformity, to allow for controlled regular motion via distraction osteogenesis, to facilitate limited compressive motion across joints or arthrodeses, or to prohibit motion absolutely.[4] They may be variably designed to be circular, monoplane, biplane, hybrid- or delta-shaped in configuration. External fixators are also advantageous in managing challenging soft tissue compromise; offloading pressure from delicate flaps or skin grafts; lengthening contracted muscular, ligamentous, or tendinous structures; and/or immobilizing severely traumatized soft tissues to allow quiescence. The use of external fixation also precludes the use of casting, and therefore eliminates the associated potential casting complications. Incisions or flaps are also easily visualized in the immediate and subacute postoperative period with the application of simple proper external fixation dressings.

In contrary, external fixation is complicated and has a steep learning curve. Knowledge of anatomic safe zones, experience, and sufficient 3-dimensional visualization are critical on the part of the surgeon. The biomechanics associated with a complicated construct must also be fully understood to prevent complications and optimize the utility of the external fixator.[1] Familiarity with minor and major postoperative complications is paramount, as these are not uncommon, even in experienced hands.[5–9] Cost may also be prohibitive, depending on the resources available, as even simple external fixators may be expensive. Moreover, patient selection is highly important as a supportive social network and frequent follow-up care is essential in the postoperative period, especially if self-directed external fixation adjustments or dressing changes are necessary.

Trauma

Acute traumatic fractures are one of the more common applications for external fixation in the lower extremity.[1,10] These fractures, depending on the mechanism of injury, may also have associated severe soft tissue compromise and may present with massive edema or fracture blisters and skin slough. With severe fracture dislocations, external fixation is sometimes used for reduction and stabilization of the affected joints and in preparation for staged reconstruction of the deformity. When bone fragments are comminuted and otherwise nonreconstructable, external fixation is used to stabilize the fragments with proximal and distal anchoring and to maintain length of the affected bone. Rigid static external fixation is highly advantageous in allowing soft tissue quiescence in the trauma setting, which is crucial to successful outcomes. Indeed, one of the primary tenets in the overall treatment of traumatic injuries includes gentle soft tissue handling and minimal soft tissue stripping, both of which are immensely easier after resolution of the massive acute reactive edema of the injured tissues (**Fig. 1**).[1,11]

Charcot Foot Neuroarthropathy and High-risk Patients

External fixation can also be advantageous in high-risk patients and severe foot and ankle pathologies. In patients with peripheral neuropathy of any cause, Charcot neuroarthropathy may develop. Through an incompletely understood pathophysiologic mechanism, the Charcot process can have catastrophic effects in the foot and lower extremity. The pathologic process fulminates in collapse of bony architecture via

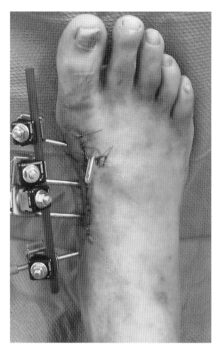

Fig. 1. A clinical picture of a monolateral uniplane external fixator for the management of a tarsometatarsal joint fracture and dislocation.

multiple severe fracture-dislocations and alterations in associated structures. As a result, the Charcot foot and ankle is significantly unstable but is masked by peripheral neuropathy through the absence of pain and proprioceptive feedback. Often, severe and recalcitrant plantar ulcerations develop in areas of high pressure; because these ulcerations may become infected and progress to contiguous osteomyelitis, appropriate treatment is of paramount importance. Chronic ulceration is the number one risk factor for the development of osteomyelitis.[12]

Successful treatment of devastating Charcot foot and/or ankle collapse and ulceration frequently warrants surgical reconstruction and stabilization of the affected areas. Although rigid internal fixation usually suffices for the treatment of simple fractures in healthy and sensate patients, patients with Charcot neuroarthropathy require so-called superconstructs to achieve rigid stabilization of pathologic osseous fragments.[13] The superconstructs include adjunctive circular external fixation,[6,14–22] plantar plates, locking plates, and/or intramedullary fixation.[6,14,19,23,24]

The use of external fixation in other high-risk patients is debatable. Patients needing revisional surgery secondary to nonunion or malunion certainly benefit from the improved stability of external fixation.[1,25,26] Patients with infected internal hardware or septic joints requiring massive bone excision and antibiotic blocks are at high risk for ulceration and further complication if the affected joint is not absolutely immobilized after surgery. These patients, who are also often diabetic, frequently benefit from external fixation for off-loading and stabilization after definitive procedures are performed on the affected joint.[1,9] Patients with diabetes and significant peripheral arterial disease may also benefit from adjunctive external fixation for ankle fractures or Charcot fracture-dislocations, because the procedures can be performed with less aggressive soft tissue dissection and smaller incisions (**Fig. 2**).[1]

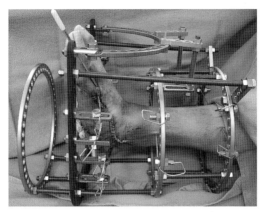

Fig. 2. A clinical picture of a circular multiplane external fixator used for the surgical management of Charcot foot reconstruction.

Plastic Reconstruction

External fixation is also an effective temporary adjunctive tool for complicated soft tissue procedures that require absolute off-loading in the postoperative period. In patients with severe soft tissue defects warranting pedicle flap coverage, hybrid external fixators can be used to off-load the posterior leg and heel and protect the flap from pressure necrosis.[27,28] These are high-risk areas for decubitus breakdown in patients recuperating in supine positions, and prevention of pressure necrosis after complex plastic procedures in these tenuous areas is paramount to their success. Likewise, patients undergoing plantar soft tissue reconstruction with local muscle flaps, rotational advancement flaps, and/or skin grafts benefit from the forced plantar off-loading of hybrid or circular external fixators.[14,28–30] Typically, external fixators applied solely for off-loading purposes are needed for shorter durations and may be removed as early as 6 to 8 weeks postoperatively,[31] whereas frames for complex deformity correction may be left in place for 8 to upwards of 30 weeks (**Fig. 3**).[5,6]

Complex Deformity Correction

The applications for external fixation in deformity correction are vast and sufficiently complex to be beyond the scope of this article. These include, but are not limited to, correction of residual clubfoot (equinocavovarus) deformity,[5,32] correction of angular deformities in any of the major osseous segments contributing to distal pathomechanics (such as tibial varus or ankle valgus),[5] arthrodeses with dynamic or sequential compression,[33–36] correction of nonreducible soft tissue equinus[1] and distraction osteogenesis (such as for congenital brachymetatarsia or infected open pilon fractures).[37,38] In addition, external fixation has been described for the open reduction and fixation of calcaneal fractures and malunions[1] and arthrodiastasis of the ankle joint to delay or obviate the need for ankle arthrodesis.[39–42] The scope of application for external fixation belies the complexity of mechanical effects that can be engineered. When directed at bone, joint, or soft tissue, compression, distraction, angular manipulation, and de novo bone formation, in unison or combination, can effect complex deformity correction with a properly designed frame.

Perioperative Nursing Considerations

In the operating room (OR), external fixation cases can be cumbersome and may require multiple sets of instruments and OR tables.[4] A skilled OR team familiar with the

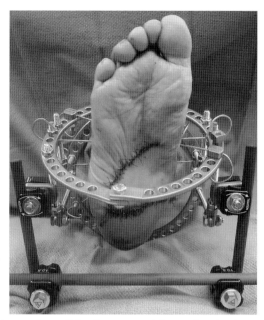

Fig. 3. A clinical picture of an off-loading external fixator for plastic surgical reconstruction of the diabetic foot.

instrumentation is crucial to the tempo of the surgery, and every setup detail is important. Proper selection of operating table so as to allow unencumbered distal intraoperative radiography saves both time and aggravation. Nearly all circular or hybrid external fixation applications in the foot and ankle requires spinal, popliteal, or general anesthesia, and the specific positioning aids must be anticipated. Conversely, external fixation removal may often be accomplished under intravenous sedation.

For most foot and ankle external fixation applications, unless specifically instructed otherwise, the patient is positioned supine with the feet located a few centimeters proximal to the end of the operating table and the patella forward.[4] Ipsilateral hip positioning is frequently necessary to maintain the distal lower extremity orthogonal to the operating table surface, and contralateral limb padding is positioned to prevent peroneal nerve damage. Adequate sterile space at the distal end of the room is essential for multiplane wire insertion. Although surgeon preference varies, often extra sterile towels are needed during the course of the case to aid in limb positioning within the circular external fixation device. OR staff must anticipate the use of intraoperative radiography and be familiar with the respective additional drapes and positioning aids required. The preferred location of the C-arm monitor ought also to be anticipated during room setup. Power instruments are crucial to the case, and extra batteries must be readily available in the room. Finally, familiarity with preferred dressings for external fixators is a crucial time-saving step at the end of each surgical case. Frequently these involve povidone-iodine solutions, multiple 4×4 gauzes, and/or elastic bandages, but may vary with surgeon preference.

SUMMARY

The applications for external fixation in the foot and ankle are wide ranging and include acute fracture immobilization, soft tissue immobilization, angular correction of congenital deformity, off-loading, arthrodesis, revisional surgery, and osseous surgery in high-risk patients. Angular relationships in the construction of external fixators are crucial, as are patient positioning and accurate medical imaging. The techniques require an experienced surgeon and surgical team.

REFERENCES

1. Molloy AP, Roche A, Narayan B. Treatment of nonunion and malunion of trauma of the foot and ankle using external fixation. Foot Ankle Clin 2009; 14:563–87.
2. Ilizarov GA. The tension stress effect on the genesis and growth of tissues: part I. The influence of stability of fixation and soft tissue preservation. Clin Orthop Relat Res 1989;238:249–81.
3. Ilizarov GA. The tension stress effect on the genesis and growth of tissues: part II. The influence of stability of fixation and soft tissue preservation. Clin Orthop Relat Res 1989;239:263–85.
4. Beaman DN, Gellman R. The basics of ring external fixator application and care. Foot Ankle Clin 2008;13:15–27.
5. Dhar S. Ilizarov external fixation in the correction of severe pediatric foot and ankle deformities. Foot Ankle Clin 2010;15:265–85.
6. Dalla Paola L, Brocco E, Ceccacci T, et al. Limb salvage in Charcot foot and ankle osteomyelitis: combined use single stage/double stage of arthrodesis and external fixation. Foot Ankle Int 2009;30:1065–70.
7. Rogers LC, Bevilacqua NJ, Frykberg RG, et al. Predictors of postoperative complications of Ilizarov external ring fixators in the foot and ankle. J Foot Ankle Surg 2007;46:372–5.
8. Wukich DK, Belczyk RJ, Burns PR, et al. Complications encountered with circular ring fixation in persons with diabetes mellitus. Foot Ankle Int 2008; 29:994–1000.
9. Zarutsky E, Rush SM, Schuberth JM. The use of circular wire external fixation in the treatment of salvage ankle arthrodesis. J Foot Ankle Surg 2005;44:22–31.
10. Tintle SM, Keeling JJ, Shawen SB. Combat foot and ankle trauma. J Surg Orthop Adv 2010;19:70–6.
11. Baumeister S, Germann G. Soft tissue coverage of the extremely traumatized foot and ankle. Foot Ankle Clin 2001;6:867–903.
12. Lavery LA, Armstrong DG, Wunderlich RP, et al. Risk factors for foot infections in individuals with diabetes. Diabetes Care 2006;29:1288–93.
13. Sammarco VJ. Superconstructs in the treatment of charcot foot deformity: plantar plating, locked plating, and axial screw fixation. Foot Ankle Clin 2009;14: 393–407.
14. Belczyk R, Ramanujam CL, Capobianco CM, et al. Combined midfoot arthrodesis, muscle flap coverage, and circular external fixation for the chronic ulcerated Charcot deformity. Foot Ankle Spec 2010;3:40–4.
15. Bevilacqua NJ, Rogers LC. Surgical management of Charcot midfoot deformities. Clin Podiatr Med Surg 2008;25:81–94.
16. Conway JD. Charcot salvage of the foot and ankle using external fixation. Foot Ankle Clin 2008;13:157–73.
17. Fabrin J, Larsen K, Holstein PE. Arthrodesis with external fixation in the unstable or misaligned Charcot ankle in patients with diabetes mellitus. Int J Low Extrem Wounds 2007;6:102–7.

18. Farber DC, Juliano PJ, Cavanagh PR, et al. Single stage correction with external fixation of the ulcerated foot in individuals with Charcot neuroarthropathy. Foot Ankle Int 2002;23:130–4.

19. Jolly GP, Zgonis T, Polyzois V. External fixation in the management of Charcot neuroarthropathy. Clin Podiatr Med Surg 2003;20:741–56.

20. Roukis TS, Zgonis T. The management of acute Charcot fracture-dislocations with the Taylor's spatial external fixation system. Clin Podiatr Med Surg 2006;23: 467–83, viii.

21. Stapleton JJ, Belczyk R, Zgonis T. Revisional Charcot foot and ankle surgery. Clin Podiatr Med Surg 2009;26:127–39.

22. Zgonis T, Roukis TS, Stapleton JJ, et al. Combined lateral column arthrodesis, medial plantar artery flap, and circular external fixation for Charcot midfoot collapse with chronic plantar ulceration. Adv Skin Wound Care 2008;21:521–5.

23. Pinzur MS. Neutral ring fixation for high-risk non-plantigrade Charcot midfoot deformity. Foot Ankle Int 2007;28:961–6.

24. Assal M, Stern R. Realignment and extended fusion with use of a medial column screw for midfoot deformities secondary to diabetic neuropathy. J Bone Joint Surg Am 2009;91:812–20.

25. Katsenis D, Bhave A, Paley D, et al. Treatment of malunion and nonunion at the site of an ankle fusion with the Ilizarov apparatus. J Bone Joint Surg Am 2005; 87:302–9.

26. Paley D, Lamm BM, Katsenis D, et al. Treatment of malunion and nonunion at the site of an ankle fusion with the Ilizarov apparatus. Surgical technique. J Bone Joint Surg Am 2006;88(Suppl 1, Pt 1):119–34.

27. Jolly GP, Zgonis T. Soft tissue reconstruction of the foot with a reverse flow sural artery neurofasciocutaneous flap. Ostomy Wound Manage 2004;50:44–9.

28. Zgonis T, Stapleton JJ, Papakostas I. Local and distant pedicle flaps for soft tissue reconstruction of the diabetic foot: a stepwise approach with the use of external fixation. In: Zgonis T, editor. Surgical reconstruction of the diabetic foot and ankle. Philadelphia: Lippincott, Williams & Wilkins; 2009. p. 179–92.

29. Belczyk R, Stapleton JJ, Zgonis T. A case report of a double advancement flap closure combined with an Ilizarov technique for the chronic plantar forefoot ulceration. Int J Low Extrem Wounds 2009;8:31–6.

30. Oznur A, Zgonis T. Closure of major diabetic foot wounds and defects with external fixation. Clin Podiatr Med Surg 2007;24:519–28.

31. Zgonis T, Stapleton JJ. Innovative techniques in preventing and salvaging neurovascular pedicle flaps in reconstructive foot and ankle surgery. Foot Ankle Spec 2008;1:97–104.

32. Ferreria RC, Costa MT. Recurrent clubfoot–Approach and treatment with external fixation. Foot Ankle Clin 2009;14:435–45.

33. Schoenhaus HD, Lam S, Treaster A, et al. Use of a small bilateral external fixator for ankle fusion. J Foot Ankle Surg 2009;48:89–92.

34. Santangelo JR, Glisson RR, Garras DN, et al. Tibiotalocalcaneal arthrodesis: a biomechanical comparison of multiplanar external fixation with intramedullary fixation. Foot Ankle Int 2008;29:936–41.

35. Calif E, Stein H, Lerner A. The Ilizarov external fixation frame in compression arthrodesis of large, weight bearing joints. Acta Orthop Belg 2004;70:51–6.

36. Zgonis T, Jolly GP. External fixation use in arthrodesis of the foot and ankle. Clin Podiatr Med Surg 2004;21:1–15.

37. Stasikelis PJ, Calhoun JH, Ledbetter BR, et al. Treatment of infected pilon nonunions with small pin fixators. Foot Ankle 1993;14:373–9.

38. Somanchi BV, Khan S. Vacuum-assisted wound closure (VAC) with simultaneous bone transport in the leg: a technical note. Acta Orthop Belg 2008;74:538–41.
39. van Valburg AA, van Roermund PM, Lammens J, et al. Can Ilizarov joint distraction delay the need for an arthrodesis of the ankle? A preliminary report. J Bone Joint Surg Br 1995;77:720–5.
40. Zgonis T, Stapleton JJ, Roukis TS. Use of circular external fixation for combined subtalar joint fusion and ankle distraction. Clin Podiatr Med Surg 2008;25:745–53.
41. Marijnissen AC, Van Roermund PM, van Melkebeek J, et al. Clinical benefit of joint distraction in the treatment of severe osteoarthritis of the ankle: proof of concept in an open prospective randomized controlled study. Arthritis Rheum 2002;46: 2893–902.
42. Ploegmakers JJ, Van Roermund PM, Van Melkebeek J, et al. Prolonged clinical benefit from joint distraction in the treatment of ankle osteoarthritis. Osteoarthr Cartil 2005;13:582–8.

Surgical Management of Diabetic Charcot Foot and Ankle Deformities

John J. Stapleton, DPM[a,b], Zacharia Facaros, DPM[c],
Vasilios D. Polyzois, MD, PhD[d], Thomas Zgonis, DPM[c],*

KEYWORDS

- Charcot neuroarthropathy • Diabetes • Deformity • Surgery
- External fixation

EPIDEMIOLOGY

Charcot neuroarthropathy (CN) is a progressive condition that involves the development of pathologic fractures, dislocations, and gross foot and ankle deformities that can lead to ulceration and infection in neuropathic patients. The development of CN is most commonly associated with diabetic peripheral neuropathy in the United States, and the surgical management of this condition is the focus of this article, but the condition may also affect any ambulatory patient with loss of protective sensation and pain insensitivity.[1,2] CN affects less than 1% of diabetic patients but occurs in up to 29% of diabetic patients with sensory neuropathy and loss of protective sensation.[1] Other causes of peripheral neuropathy and progression to CN that have been documented include alcoholism, chemotherapy agents, congenital insensitivity to pain, leprosy, syphilis, and renal dialysis.[3] This pathologic process, which occurs most commonly in the foot and ankle, can be idiopathic, secondary to acute trauma, previous surgery, previous pedal amputations, or can be caused by repetitive microinjury.[1,4] Continued ambulation once the acute CN process has been initiated results in progressive collapse and deformity. Severe deformities can affect the patient's ambulatory status and, when associated with instability, ulceration, and/or infection, there is a greater risk of a major limb amputation.[5] This article discusses the role of surgical management of a diabetic Charcot foot and ankle

[a] Foot and Ankle Surgery, VSAS Orthopaedics, Allentown, PA, USA
[b] Penn State College of Medicine, Hershey, PA, USA
[c] Division of Podiatric Medicine and Surgery, Department of Orthopaedics, University of Texas Health Science Center at San Antonio, 7703 Floyd Curl Drive, MSC 7776, San Antonio, TX 78229, USA
[d] Orthopaedic Traumatology, KAT General Hospital, Athens, Greece
* Corresponding author.
E-mail address: zgonis@uthscsa.edu

Perioperative Nursing Clinics 6 (2011) 67–74
doi:10.1016/j.cpen.2010.10.011
1556-7931/11/$ – see front matter © 2011 Elsevier Inc. All rights reserved.
periopnursing.theclinics.com

deformity and emphasizes the role of a knowledgeable multidisciplinary team to better treat and educate patients who suffer from CN.

INDICATIONS/CONTRAINDICATIONS OF SURGERY

The goal of surgical management of a diabetic Charcot foot and ankle deformity is to achieve a stable foot, without any infection, that will allow for an ambulatory status when supplemented with custom foot wear, orthoses, or bracing. Not all Charcot foot and ankle deformities require surgical intervention. Understanding the criteria for performing surgery, along with the contraindications, is important to avoid potential complications from early surgical intervention.

Criteria for surgical management of a diabetic Charcot foot and ankle deformity include, but are not limited to, unstable midfoot deformity, with or without ulceration; stable midfoot deformity with ulceration or preulcerative lesion; unstable rearfoot and ankle deformities, with or without ulceration; stable rearfoot and ankle deformities not amenable to custom bracing or with ulceration; acute CN resulting in soft tissue compromise; and CN deformity with underlying acute/chronic osteomyelitis. In addition, to be considered a surgical candidate, the patient must have been ambulatory before the Charcot event; must have an absence of arterial insufficiency that must be evident or addressed before surgical intervention to ensure adequate perfusion to the foot; must be medically stable and comorbidities be optimized before surgery, unless associated with a limb and/or life-threatening infection; must display compliance and the necessary cognitive function to understand the severity of the condition to prevent postoperative complication and address any detrimental psychosocial factors before considering elective reconstructive surgery.

Contraindications for surgery include, but are not limited to, the following: bedridden patient before the Charcot event, medically unstable patient, arterial insufficiency that is not amenable to intervention to improve tissue perfusion, untreated osteomyelitis, and soft tissue infection or persistent recurrent infections. Relative contraindications include, but are not limited, to an acute CN with no soft tissue compromise, morbid obesity, severe tobacco use, venous insufficiency, lymphedema, poor nutritional status, retinopathy-induced blindness, and end-stage renal disease.

PERIOPERATIVE CONSIDERATIONS

Multiple and variable case scenarios exist for the surgical management of Charcot foot and ankle deformities. The approach to the overall management of the diabetic Charcot foot and/or ankle deformity must address multiple presenting factors in conjunction with a thorough evaluation and intense medical management of the patients' comorbidities. Surgical procedures vary greatly and are dependent on the overall clinical presentation. Some cases are complicated by the presence of infection, which poses great risk for limb loss. The most difficult Charcot foot and ankle deformities to manage are those with significant soft tissue loss and deep infection.[6,7] The scenario is usually further complicated by the patients typically being morbidly obese and possibly having vascular insufficiency requiring revascularization before considering a Charcot reconstruction. Because operative intervention may involve multiple complicating issues, a stepwise rationale approach with appropriate procedure selection based on these inherent factors with a strong understanding of the timing of surgery is essential for the patient's successful outcome.

As with any Charcot reconstructive case, a thorough history and physical examination, vascular assessment, review of precipitating events, pertinent radiographs and imaging studies, and laboratory testing serve as the foundation of surgical preparation or for establishing which patients are not surgical candidates . Careful preoperative evaluation and patient selection is fundamental to reducing the risks associated with reconstructive surgery. Neglecting issues such as patient compliance and psychosocial issues only leads to further complications regardless of the surgical plan and capabilities of the treating team. Awareness of patient-related variables that may increase the risks of complications should allow for better preoperative planning and overall management of the patient.

The overall goals and a treatment plan with a time frame need to be established early so that all team members are working efficiently and toward the same goal. The critical role of the nursing staff is to understand each team member's role and to help coordinate and facilitate this dynamic relationship to achieve successful outcomes for the patient.

Should the patient elect to undergo lower limb reconstruction, the surgical team must attempt to anticipate perioperative and long-term postoperative problems and have services in place before any issues become unmanageable. Some of the complex case presentations that perioperative nursing staff need to be familiar with may include, but are not limited to, the following: patients with chronic ulceration as a result of a Charcot deformity and questionable infection have to be screened for methicillin-resistant *Staphylococcus aureus* (MRSA) colonization; patients with CN and deep infection typically require placement of a peripherally inserted central catheter line for long-term parenteral antibiotic therapy; patients with CN typically require inpatient medical management by internal medicine along with multiple subspecialty services; cardiology consultation may be required if there is significant history for coronary artery disease and/or risk factors for myocardial infarction and for risk stratification when reconstructive surgery is considered; vascular surgery consultation is required in the presence of arterial insufficiency. Angiograms are typically performed by the interventional radiologists or vascular surgery service in patients who require revascularization and/or soft tissue reconstruction with a pedicle flap; nephrology consultation is required to continue and coordinate renal dialysis in patients with acute renal failure and/or end-stage renal disease who are dependent on dialysis; endocrinologist consultation is also important to help establish better glycemic control throughout the perioperative period and to provide long-term follow-up care; diabetic nurse educators are required to ensure that patients comprehend and are knowledgeable in the overall management of their disease; activity orders have to be clarified and documented by the nursing staff to avoid potential complications. Physical therapists and physiatrists, along with the surgeon, are required in determining rehabilitation needs; deep vein thrombosis (DVT) prophylaxis is recommended in this population secondary to the inherent risk factors and mobility constraints that are usually encountered. The method of DVT prophylaxis is often dependent on the patient's renal function, past medical history, and need for further staged surgical procedures; consents for blood transfusions are often needed because these patients are usually chronically anemic and significant blood loss can be encountered with major reconstructive procedures; dieticians and nutritionists are used for meal recommendations and to educate the patient in proper long-term eating habits; a smoking cessation program needs to be established for those patients who are dependent on and/or addicted to tobacco products; psychologists and social workers are needed when psychosocial factors have to be addressed. Patients are typically encountered with loss of employment, long-term disability, and/or career changes as a result of their condition; and time must be spent with discharge planning to be certain that all postoperative orders and follow-up appointments are clarified and comprehended by the patient and family. Patients who are being transferred to other subacute, rehabilitation, and/or extended health care facilities need to be made aware of all orders before discharge to be certain that available resources are in place for the necessary postoperative care, including long-term footwear and bracing.

Charcot Deformity with Ulceration and/or Infection

Ulceration and infection are commonly encountered in the Charcot foot.[8] Deep soft tissue infection resulting in osteomyelitis further complicates the clinical case and overall management of a Charcot deformity. Several publications have focused on differentiating CN from osteomyelitis.[9,10] The clinical concern is not differentiating between the 2 but whether the Charcot deformity and dystrophic bone is further complicated with osteomyelitis when an ulcer is present. Charcot deformities with ulcerations that display clinical evidence of infection marked by purulent or malodorous drainage can be assumed to be complicated with a deep infection. Ulcerations that clinically present with bone exposure are also treated for osteomyelitis. Typically, the patient is initially brought to the operating room to perform an ulcer excision with incision and drainage and obtainment of deep soft cultures along with bone biopsy and culture to guide treatment. The patient is then started on empirical parenteral antibiotics by the infectious disease service, which is later tailored based on the clinical presentation along with the intraoperative culture and sensitivity results. Positive bone cultures should be treated with surgical osseous resection if feasible, along with a recommended course of intravenous antibiotics to treat the presumed pathogen. Staged procedures are typically required to achieve osseous resection for management of osteomyelitis and Charcot deformity correction. Typically, a delayed fusion, approximately 6 to 8 weeks or longer after medical and surgical management of the deep infection has been performed, is required to salvage a septic Charcot deformity. Often, external fixation is used in these cases to avoid internal fixation with the history of infection.[11] In addition, plastic surgical reconstruction is commonly required to achieve delayed wound closure.[12]

Unstable Rocker-bottom Charcot Midfoot Deformity

Determining instability in a Charcot midfoot deformity can be more difficult during physical examination, as opposed to rearfoot and ankle deformities that display obvious unstable deformities. In rare cases, frank instability is appreciated on clinical examination, but this is not the common clinical scenario. More often, the patients display a rocker-bottom deformity, medial or lateral column collapse, forefoot abduction, or adduction that appears clinically rigid and stable. However, subtle joint instability is often apparent, especially when soft tissue compromise is present. The authors typically use a combination of serial radiographs that are taken non–weight bearing and compared with weight-bearing images to determine the presence of joint subluxation and collapse. In addition, computed tomography is beneficial for determining the presence of osseous consolidation and bone bridging across the Charcot midfoot deformity. Determining the presence of joint instability becomes important when considering surgical intervention, especially if a simple ostectomy is being considered. Often, ostectomy procedures are performed in elderly patients and in patients with multiple comorbidities who are not considered stable for an extensive surgical reconstruction. The problem arises when an ostectomy is performed on an unstable Charcot midfoot deformity or if an ostectomy will compromise joint stability by removing the osseous bridging that was developed around the affected fractures and joint subluxations. Surgical ostectomy should be reserved for truly stable Charcot midfoot deformities that do not display further joint subluxation on weight-bearing radiographs and would not be compromised by performing the procedure. Charcot midfoot deformities with joint instability are best treated with extended joint arthrodesis procedures to prevent later collapse and future complications. They may be surgically corrected with internal fixation, external fixation, or a combination of both.[13–15] External fixation is typically used in patients with poor bone stock, previous osseous resection, previous history of infection, and/or who display a poor soft tissue envelope. Internal fixation is typically used when reasonable bone stock is present along with a good soft tissue envelope. Recently, advances in internal fixation in plate designs and locking plate capability have offered further options to osseous reconstruction for Charcot midfoot deformities.[16]

Operating Room Setup

Preparing the operating room is a task typically performed by the perioperative nurse, circulating nurse, the surgeon's assistant, and the surgical technician. Instrumentation and table setups are more efficient if the surgeon works regularly with familiar staff, especially in complex case scenarios. Charcot reconstructive cases can require abundant trays and equipment that are used through various portions of the procedure. If a surgeon discusses in advance his protocol for table setup and the need for particular equipment that is not routinely supplied in basic orthopaedic trays, operating time is reduced. Once the operating room is prepared and all equipment is available, the perioperative nurse and anesthesiology care provider transport the patient to the operating room on a stretcher and assist the patient to transfer to the operative bed. All nonoperative extremities are padded with foam and secured. The perioperative nurse assists the anesthesiology care provider during the initial induction. A Foley catheter may be inserted according to the discretion of the anesthesiologist and surgeon. A bump is typically positioned under the ipsilateral hip if the patient is supine on the operating table to place the foot in a rectus position. Positioning of the limb is critical and final patient positioning should be assessed by the surgeon before skin preparation. The surgeon must consider surgical exposure and incision placement, intraoperative fluoroscopy views that need to be obtained, and alignment of the leg for osseous corrections, intramedullary nailing and/or placement of external fixation devices. If a tourniquet is used, cast padding is wrapped around the thigh or calf and an appropriately sized cuff is placed. The exception to this is patients who underwent recent vascular surgical intervention. In these cases, an Esmarch bandage should be available on the field and may be required to assist in local hemostasis during portions of the procedures. A nonadherent drape is then be placed over the tourniquet if used to maintain a clean surgical site. The electrocautery is grounded on a clean, intact skin area on the thigh or abdomen. If the patient has no signs of peripheral vascular disease or any other contraindications for the use of compression stockings, a pneumatic sequential compression device is applied on the nonsurgical lower extremity to further prevent the incidence of DVT and pulmonary embolism in the postoperative period.

The perioperative nurse performs a team timeout to confirm the patient's identity, verify the procedure and surgical site(s), and verify that required equipment is available before beginning a surgical preparation. The surgical preparation is performed following recommended operative and practice guidelines established for the hospital. The perioperative nurse, along with the scrub technician, prepares the sterile surgical field. Surgical drapes that are applied should allow exposure of the knee to facilitate correct positioning during deformity correction.

Standard basic orthopaedic trays that also include curved and straight osteotomes, flexible chisels, bone hooks, distractors, lamina spreaders, large and small Steinmann pins, sagittal saws, and wire drivers are used to perform joint resection(s) and/or osteotomies. As mentioned previously, operative trays and additional tables should be prepared for the equipment to be used to apply internal fixation, external fixation, and/or intramedullary nailing. C-arm for intraoperative imaging should be draped and positioned on the opposite side to the operative limb. A radiolucent table is necessary to obtain alignment radiographs because limb position is paramount to the Charcot reconstruction surgery. A basic plastic or neurosurgery tray with fine and more delicate instrumentation may also be required if a plastic surgery procedure is needed for soft tissue coverage in conjunction with the Charcot reconstruction.

Electrocautery should be established for each patient. Often, diabetic patients undergoing Charcot reconstruction are also cardiac patients with pacemakers. The use of a magnet and/or bipolar cautery may be warranted in these select cases and this should be discussed with the surgeon and the anesthesiologist to prevent cardiac complications.

It is common for bone grafting to be either autogenous and/or allogenic in Charcot reconstructive surgery. Typical donor sites, such as the ipsilateral or contralateral iliac crest, need to be prepared and separate instrumentation set up for harvest so that 2 surgical teams can work simultaneously, if available. If orthobiologics, such as allogenic bone grafting, bone morphogenic proteins, and platelet-rich and -poor plasma are to be used, they should be readily available in the room. In addition, it is important to be knowledgeable in the preparation and allocated exposure times for such products so they can be prepared in advance to reduce operative time.

It is paramount for the surgeon and perioperative nurse to discuss the specifics of the surgical instrumentation that will be needed, orthobiologics to be used, suture supplies and/or use of intraoperative imaging before the surgery is initiated. Postoperative dressing materials may also be available and ready in the room to further prevent prolonged operating time and anesthesia recovery. An operating room that is set up with the necessary instrumentation greatly facilitates the surgery in these patients at high risk (**Figs. 1** and **2**).

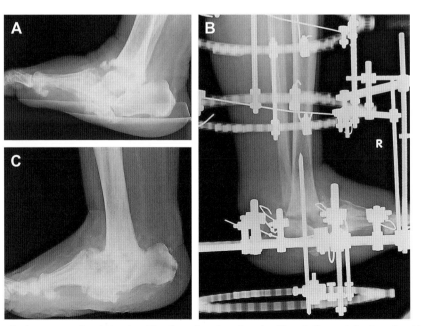

Fig. 1. A preoperative lateral ankle view showing the significant Charcot foot and ankle collapse (A) treated with a total talectomy and tibiocalcaneal arthrodesis with an Ilizarov circular external fixator (B). Final radiographic view showing the arthrodesis site (C).

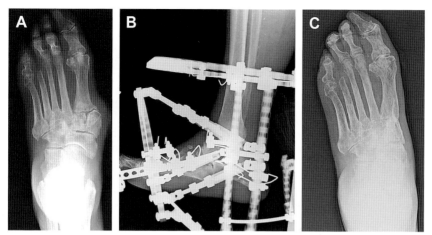

Fig. 2. A preoperative anteroposterior foot view showing the significant Charcot foot collapse (*A*) treated with a medial column arthrodesis and a modified circular external fixator (*B*). Final radiographic view showing the arthrodesis site (*C*).

Postoperative Care and Rehabilitation

After surgery, the patient is typically hospitalized for a period of time that is dependent on the staged procedures and overall medical status of the patient. When patients are medically optimized, they are usually transferred to an extended care facility until they are able to follow postoperative and rehabilitation orders. During this period, the operative limb is kept elevated, decubitus wound precautions need to be implemented, and the patient is typically on a non–weight-bearing status to the affected extremity or confined to a wheelchair in certain clinical scenarios.

DVT prophylaxis is usually started on the first postoperative day. The patient is initially instructed by the physical therapist to perform exercises if permitted by the surgeon while in bed. Training with a walker or crutches to be strictly non–weight bearing is common once the patient is allowed to transfer from the bed to a sitting position. This training can involve a lot of effort and time by the patient and the therapist, especially if external fixation devices were used in surgery because they tend to be heavy and bulky. Dressing changes are dependent on the procedure performed. Patients with Charcot-induced ulcerations often require local wound care and frequent dressing changes or application of negative-pressure wound therapy. Patients who underwent closure of soft tissue defects with a random or pedicle flap typically require close observation to ensure that the flap is viable and not compromised with hematoma and/or venous congestion.

In general, the patient on discharge is followed every 10 to 14 days after surgery. The patient is usually kept strictly non–weight bearing for the postoperative period. The authors do not advocate early weight bearing for the diabetic patient with dense peripheral neuropathy. If an external fixator was used, the patient does not routinely care for pin and/or wire sites; however, this is still the surgeon's preference. The external fixation device is then removed in the operating room under intravenous sedation and local anesthesia and based on the procedure(s) selected for the patients. After the external fixator removal, the patient is usually kept non–weight bearing for an additional 2 to 6 weeks using a lower extremity fiberglass cast or an offloading boot. The patient is then progressed to partial and full weight bearing with the use of therapeutic shoes and bracing, as needed, by an experienced health care provider.

SUMMARY

A stepwise proactive approach to avoiding complications associated with a Charcot foot and ankle deformity is essential for functional limb preservation. A multidisciplinary team consisting of surgical, medical, nursing, and nutritional disciplines with knowledge and experience in Charcot deformities is needed to adequately manage this devastating disease process. Understanding the indications for surgery, timing of surgery, and staging of surgical procedures is paramount to a successful outcome and the overall perioperative management of the patient. The goal for operating on the Charcot foot is to provide the patient with a limb that is stable, mechanically sound, and resistant to further breakdown while resuming an ambulatory status to improve their overall health.

REFERENCES

1. Frykberg RG, Zgonis T, Armstrong DG, et al. Diabetic foot disorders. A clinical practice guideline (2006 revision). J Foot Ankle Surg 2006;45(Suppl 5):S1–66.
2. van der Ven A, Chapman CB, Bowker JH. Charcot neuroarthropathy of the foot and ankle. J Am Acad Orthop Surg 2009;17(9):562–71.
3. Shibuya N, La Fontaine J, Frania SJ. Alcohol-induced neuroarthropathy in the foot: a case series and review of literature. J Foot Ankle Surg 2008;47(2):118–24.
4. Crews RT, Wrobel JS. Physical management of the Charcot foot. Clin Podiatr Med Surg 2008;25(1):71–9.
5. Cavanagh PR, Bus SA. Off-loading the diabetic foot for ulcer prevention and healing. J Am Podiatr Med Assoc 2010;100(5):360–8.
6. Zgonis T, Jolly GP, Buren BJ, et al. Diabetic foot infections and antibiotic therapy. Clin Podiatr Med Surg 2003;20:655–69.
7. Zgonis T, Stapleton JJ, Roukis TS. A stepwise approach to the surgical management of severe diabetic foot infections. Foot Ankle Spec 2008;1(1):46–53.
8. Sohn MW, Stuck RM, Pinzur M, et al. Lower-extremity amputation risk after Charcot arthropathy and diabetic foot ulcer. Diabetes Care 2010;33(1):98–100.
9. Sella EJ, Grosser DM. Imaging modalities of the diabetic foot. Clin Podiatr Med Surg 2003;20(4):729–40.
10. Boc SF, Brazzo K, Lavian D, et al. Acute Charcot foot changes versus osteomyelitis: does Tc-99m HMPAO labeled leukocytes scan differentiate? J Am Podiatr Med Assoc 2001;91(7):365–8.
11. Jolly GP, Zgonis T, Polyzois V. External fixation in the management of Charcot neuroarthropathy. Clin Podiatr Med Surg 2003;20(4):741–56.
12. Zgonis T, Roukis TS, Stapleton JJ, et al. Combined lateral column arthrodesis, medial plantar artery flap, and circular external fixation for Charcot midfoot collapse with chronic plantar ulceration. Adv Skin Wound Care 2008;21(11):521–5.
13. Zgonis T, Roukis TS, Lamm BM. Charcot foot and ankle reconstruction: current thinking and surgical approaches. Clin Podiatr Med Surg 2007;24(3):505–17.
14. Farber DC, Juliano PJ, Cavanagh PR, et al. Single stage correction with external fixation of the ulcerated foot in individuals with Charcot neuroarthropathy. Foot Ankle Int 2002;23(2):130–4.
15. Grant WP, Garcia-Lavin SE, Sabo RT, et al. A retrospective analysis of 50 consecutive Charcot diabetic salvage reconstructions. J Foot Ankle Surg 2009;48(1):30–8.
16. Capobianco CM, Stapleton JJ, Zgonis T. The role of an extended medial column arthrodesis for Charcot midfoot neuroarthropathy. Diabetic Foot & Ankle 2010;1:1–5.

Postoperative Complications in Foot and Ankle Reconstruction

Zacharia Facaros, DPM, Steven P. Kissel, DPM,
Michael G. Palladino, DPM, Thomas Zgonis, DPM*

KEYWORDS

• Postoperative complications • Foot • Ankle • Infection
• Surgery

In the preoperative setting and evaluation, a lack of proper planning and concrete diagnosis or incorrect surgical implication may produce unfavorable results for both the surgeon and the patient. Although many complications are unpredictable, most can be anticipated when accurately considering the patient's overall presentation and the planned procedures.[1]

The goal of foot and ankle reconstructive surgery is to provide pain relief from the debilitating deformity and restore function by achieving a plantigrade weight-bearing lower extremity. Before surgery is offered, it is imperative that all treatment options are discussed, with an interval of conservative or nonsurgical treatment modalities, if applicable. On surgical preparation, meticulous detailing of all risks, benefits, and possible complications requires discussion and emphasis should be placed on particular occurrences for specific procedures. This discussion should take place with the patients and their families, friends, or significant others who will be present during the patients' healing period. It is critical that the patients have someone who is supportive and able to provide assistance when needed, specifically so in the acute postoperative setting when mobility is limited.

The procedure consent form requires the incorporation of the specified diagnosis, the names of the surgeon and those in the surgical team performing the procedure, an exact description of the planned procedure, and a list of possible complications that may present. Depending on the procedure, possible common impediments may be anticipated in some cases. The surgeon-patient relationship must be a trusting and open communicative one to maximize the healing period for a smooth and safe

Division of Podiatric Medicine and Surgery, Department of Orthopaedics, University of Texas Health Science Center at San Antonio, 7703 Floyd Curl Drive/MCS 7776, San Antonio, TX 78229, USA
* Corresponding author.
E-mail address: zgonis@uthscsa.edu

Perioperative Nursing Clinics 6 (2011) 75–88
doi:10.1016/j.cpen.2010.10.002
1556-7931/11/$ – see front matter © 2011 Elsevier Inc. All rights reserved.

transition back to full recovery. Most complications in foot and ankle surgery occur postoperatively, causing significant costs to patients, hospitals, and health insurers.[2]

With an increasing percentage of elderly patients who are not only burdened by pain from acute musculoskeletal conditions but also expected to stay active longer than did previous generations, the foot and ankle surgeon will continue to see an increase in the number of patients with neglected deformities and comorbidities that contribute to an unfavorable healing potential. Several conditions exist that require reconstructive surgery, some of which include severe sprains, ruptures, dislocations, and fractures, whereas a separate subset of patients present with complications stemming from diabetes mellitus, renal disease, and Charcot neuroarthropathy.

This article addresses some of the fundamental complications in the postoperative setting, such as management of uncontrolled pain, deep vein thrombosis (DVT), pulmonary embolism (PE), infection, and common rehabilitation obstacles.

PAIN MANAGEMENT

Pain, nausea, and vomiting are common complaints after surgical anesthesia, especially when general anesthesia is implemented.[3] One of the obligatory criteria for considering surgical intervention is a constant level of pain endured on a daily basis. It is mandatory to discuss the anticipated pain that may result postoperatively, and the patient must be informed if there may always be a certain level of pain or discomfort, regardless of the action taken. Proper postoperative pain management is an extremely significant phase of the healing period.

The goals in achieving successful pain management are to minimize pain, enhance the quality of recovery, and promote a quick and safe return to normal activities of daily living. Acute postoperative pain from ambulatory surgery tends to be undertreated, and the negative effect of such surgery causes disruption in the peripheral and central nervous system, potentially leading to the development of chronic pain.[4,5] It has been documented that acute pain results in various physiologic changes, having important effects on the patient's clinical course, and unrelieved pain may cause adverse effects on more than one body system, particularly in high-risk surgical patients.[6,7] For instance, severe postoperative pain and increased levels of sympathetic activity may cause spasms in arterial inflow and venous emptying and are also common reasons for delays in hospital discharge and unanticipated hospital admissions, which, in turn, impairs the cost-effectiveness of ambulatory surgery.[8,9] Adequate pain relief after surgery can increase mobility and expedite a patient's return to normal function, providing earlier return to work and a psychological benefit.[10]

Pain is not homogeneous and usually comprises 3 categories: physiologic, inflammatory, and neuropathic.[11] Multiple mechanisms contribute to pain, each of which is subject to or an expression of neural plasticity, which is the capacity of neurons to change their function, chemical profile, or structure.[11] Acute pain results from mechanically, chemically, or thermally induced damage to tissue integrity, all of which may be encountered by the patient during surgery. An assortment of chemicals released by damaged cells in response to tissue injury and local inflammation, including histamine, bradykinin, prostaglandins, serotonin, substance P, acetylcholine, and leukotrienes, further sensitize nociceptors to other noxious stimuli, sequentially leading to the aforementioned neuronal plasticity.[11] Further discussion on the cellular and molecular mechanism of pain is beyond the scope of this article, and the next objective is to discuss how pain may be minimized and properly managed.

Reconstructive foot and ankle procedures require postoperative pain management to provide analgesia beyond 24 hours. Numerous patients, especially the elderly, may have several comorbid conditions and multiple sources of pain, including musculoskeletal and neuropathic pain, which the surgeon must help manage in the postoperative setting. Prescribers must accurately select an analgesic regimen that can control pain while minimizing the side effects and interactions with any concurrent medication. The selection of an accurate regimen represents a challenge for the surgeon because there are often overlapping complex conditions with multiple causes of pain. The goal must be to provide pain management that optimizes efficacy and safety and is also simple and easy for the patient to use. Before surgery discussion, a dialogue between the patient and the surgeon must transpire to evaluate the patient's pain tolerance, history of complications or drug abuse in related instances, and expectations in the short- and long-term settings.

Surgical anesthesia is a fundamental contributing factor and is directly related to the magnitude of the postoperative pain. Choosing the anesthetic technique for surgery is the decision of the anesthesiologist, and both the patient and surgeon are consulted as to which technique best suits the safety and ideal preference for a clean and uneventful procedure. Regardless of whether the surgery transpires in the inpatient or outpatient setting, the goals of anesthesia are patient safety and analgesia, optimal operating conditions, control of intra- and postoperative pain, and avoidance of general endotracheal anesthesia and its inherent risk factors, when applicable.[12] Certain situations require administration of general anesthesia; however, regional anesthetic techniques have more opportunity for success in foot and ankle surgery because of the peripheral location of the surgical site and the opportunity to temporarily anesthetize sensory and motor nerve pathways.[12] General and regional anesthesia options have their respective positions in foot and ankle surgery, with few instances allowing for adequate coverage from a single local anesthesia. Many patients requiring foot and ankle reconstruction have predisposing comorbidities, such as diabetes mellitus, kidney disease, coronary artery disease, and obesity, each maintaining further inherent risks, which further contribute to the anesthetic cause.

Regional anesthesia consisting of intravenous (IV) sedation with a peripherally placed nerve block is typically implemented for effective intra- and postoperative surgical pain management. Regional anesthetic techniques can be further divided into those performed centrally and peripherally. The central techniques pertain to the neuroaxial blocks (epidural anesthesia, spinal anesthesia), and the peripheral techniques can be further divided into plexus blocks and single nerve blocks. Medication for regional anesthesia may be given as a single shot or continuously over a prolonged period through a catheter.[13,14] Furthermore, regional anesthesia can be provided by injecting local anesthetics directly into the veins of the patient's arm while impeding the venous flow by a tourniquet, referred to as a Bier block.[15]

These modes of anesthesia are versatile in that any foot and ankle surgical procedure may be effectively covered. The anesthesiologist and surgeon must have a working knowledge of the involved anatomy, local anesthetic pharmacology, and technical expertise to safely and properly perform anesthesia and avoid insufficient anesthesia and potential toxicity. IV sedation during block placement provides anxiolysis, amnesia, and induced sleepiness.[16,17] Again, various sedative agents may be used depending on the patient's medical history, surgical procedure, and preference of the anesthesiologist. Benzodiazepines are ideal because they provide amnestic and anxiolytic properties, as well as raise the seizure threshold, providing an additional margin of safety in case of inadvertent local anesthetic toxicity.[16,17] Barbiturates and opioids may also be given; opioids are mainly used as supplements to the barbiturates and benzodiazepines.[16,17] There are several medications within these categories, all used for their adjunctive ability for sedation, the commonly implemented drugs being midazolam, propofol, etomidate, fentanyl, and pentobarbital sodium.[16,17]

The nerve supply to the foot and ankle originates in the anterior divisions of the spinal nerve roots of L4-S3 in the lumbosacral spine. The leg may be divided into 4 respective compartments, whereas 3 compartments run the entire length of the foot and 5 compartments are confined to the forefoot. The hindfoot has a single calcaneal deep compartment. The anatomic mapping of nerve distribution in relation to the adjacent osseous, tendinous, ligamentous, and soft tissue supporting structures is paramount when planning a peripheral nerve block. Depending on the surgical procedure, select nerves may be technically isolated for blockade; however, foot and ankle surgeons often have used multiple types of accurately placed and well-executed peripheral nerve blocks, targeting the popliteal sciatic, common peroneal, and saphenous nerves for both pre- and postoperative pain control.[18] These blocks are based on multifactorial considerations, depending on the psychological makeup of the patients and their relative tolerance of pain, the site and nature of the operation, and the amount of surgical trauma anticipated.[18] This article focuses on nerve blocks situated at and below the ankle.

The ankle block consists of anesthetizing 6 nerves, including the medial and intermediate dorsal cutaneous branches of the superficial peroneal nerve, deep peroneal nerve, posterior tibial nerve, sural nerve, and saphenous nerve. The superficial peroneal, sural, and saphenous nerves are cutaneous extensions of the sciatic and femoral nerves. The superficial peroneal nerve perforates the deep fascia on the anterior aspect of the distal two-thirds of the leg and then travels subcutaneously, innervating the dorsum of the foot, except for the intermetatarsal and digital space between the hallux and the second toe. The sural nerve is a pure sensory nerve that is formed from the branches of the common peroneal and tibial nerves, descending into the posterior compartment of the leg and entering the foot behind the lateral malleolus and anterior to the Achilles tendon. It provides innervation to the lateral aspect of the ankle and foot. The saphenous nerve is the sensory terminal branch of the femoral nerve and becomes subcutaneous at the medial side of the knee joint, following the great saphenous vein to the medial malleolus. It innervates the medial portion of the leg to the medial malleolus and below the ankle to the midfoot region. The deep peroneal nerve courses down the anterior aspect of the interosseous membrane of the leg and proceeds to a point midway between the malleoli, where it divides into its terminal branches, and onto the dorsum of the foot. It innervates the extensors of the toes as well as the region between the hallux and the second toe. The posterior tibial nerve travels through the lower leg in conjunction with the posterior tibial artery, down the posterior aspect of the calf, and then moves medially and between the Achilles tendon and the malleolus. It divides into the medial and lateral plantar nerves at the junction of the skin where the plantar sole and proximal-medial heel meet, innervating the ankle, heel, and sole of the foot.

The Mayo block is typically used for procedures involving forefoot reconstruction of the first metatarsal and hallux. The structures include the medial dorsal cutaneous, deep peroneal, saphenous, and medial plantar nerves. The medial dorsal cutaneous nerve has a terminal branch, the first dorsal digital proper nerve that extends medially along the big toe, which thus requires blockade. For reconstructive procedures involving the toes, the digital block focuses on the terminal nerve extensions known as the dorsal and plantar digital proper nerves. If anesthesia is required more proximally, the dorsal and plantar digital common nerves, which traverse the metatarsals but not, however, to the medial or lateral aspects of the first and fifth metatarsals, respectively, may be blocked as well.

Numerous local anesthetic agents are used in peripheral nerve block injections; the choice of the agent depends on many factors, such as the desired time of onset and the duration of anesthesia. Esters and amides constitute local anesthetic agents. Esters are formed from an alcohol and acid by the removal of water, whereas amides are formed from an acid by replacing the hydroxide group with an amide group.[19] Esters are metabolized in the blood stream by pseudocholinesterase and, thus, are more quickly detoxified but display a high potential for hypersensitivity. Amides are detoxified in the liver, and thus, their effects are prolonged. When choosing a local anesthetic for injection, it is imperative that the patient's medical history and known allergies to both food and medications are reviewed. Knowledge of the toxic dose of the agent is essential as well. Some additional guidelines for local anesthesia include agent concentration and effect, volume used in relation to nerve diameter, anesthesia time lag before onset, epinephrine effect when not contraindicated, and avoiding infiltration into an infected or traumatized area.

The 2 local anesthetic drug agents that are frequently used in foot and ankle surgery are lidocaine (Xylocaine) and bupivacaine (Marcaine).[19,20] When considering which agent to implement and how much, the dosages are routinely based on an average healthy 70-kg man or 60-kg woman. In patients with significant health issues and comorbidities, the precautions must be carefully reviewed and a proper injection technique must be maintained to avoid intravascular infusion. Lidocaine is an ester with the duration of onset involving 1 to 2 hours and a maximum plain dosage of 4.5 mg/kg (300 mg maximum dose), whereas the dosage with epinephrine is 7 mg/kg (500 mg maximum dose).[21] Bupivacaine is an amide with duration of onset involving 3 to 12 hours and a maximum plain dosage being 2 mg/kg (175 mg maximum dose), whereas the dosage with epinephrine is 3 mg/kg (225 mg maximum dose).[19–24] Furthermore, knowledge of the appropriate adjustments to anesthetic doses must be meticulously considered in the infant, child, elderly, and debilitated patients. Numerous investigators have discussed their preference of local anesthetic agents and the recommended dosages,[19–24] but ultimately, the level of experience and comfort regarding both the injection technique and the medication used play major roles in the frequency of use.

Pain is a leading cause of morbidity, and management requires a critical tapering of pharmacologic therapy to promote a healthy and expedited recovery. Various oral medications may be dispensed for control; some medications have been discontinued because of unwanted side effects, whereas others are preferred because of anecdotal evidence within a surgeon's experience. Over recent years, the US Food and Drug Administration has incorporated boxed warnings on all prescription nonselective nonsteroidal antiinflammatory drugs (NSAIDs) and cyclooxygenase-2 (COX-2)-specific inhibitors, both traditionally used first choices for pain management. These drugs have been associated with cardiovascular, gastrointestinal, and cutaneous adverse events and should be used with caution when long-term pharmacologic treatment is sought.[25] An alternative to prescribing COX-2-selective drugs is to combine nonselective NSAIDs with a potentially gastrointestinal protective drug, such as proton pump inhibitors, H_2 receptor antagonists, or a prostaglandin analogue.[25,26] Acetaminophen is a well-established, effective, and well-tolerated agent in the management of mild to moderate pain.[25,26] It has none of the renal or cardiovascular side effects that are characteristic of antiinflammatory drugs and can be used as a substitute to NSAID therapy.

Acetaminophen in combination with codeine is also a popular analgesic treatment option, shown to be an improvement compared with acetaminophen alone.[25,26]

The opioid class of drugs for both acute and chronic pain management is generally reserved for moderate to severe levels of pain. These medications are often implemented in the postoperative setting as well; however, their side effects include constipation and dry mouth, and first-time users may experience nausea and/or vomiting.[25–27] Nausea and dizziness often resolve if the patient is able to persist with the medication, whereas somnolence is another common symptom experience early in the treatment phase.[25–27] In addition, the risk of developing chemical dependence and/or addiction should always be contemplated.

In a hospital setting, patient-controlled analgesia (PCA) refers to an electronically controlled infusion pump that delivers a prescribed amount of IV analgesic to the patient when a button is activated. PCA is primarily administered via IV or epidural administration routes and is commonly and effectively used to manage acute pain.[28] However, PCA-related errors are particularly dangerous because the medications used (ie, opioids) have narrow therapeutic indexes, and relatively small mistakes in dosing concentrations can potentially lead to serious or even fatal consequences.[29]

The term balanced analgesia describes the use of more than one analgesic modality or agent, with the aim of achieving enhanced analgesic efficacy and reduced side effects. Effective pain management is needed for elimination of pain or at least its reduction to a tolerable level so as to restore physical, psychological, and social functioning in the postoperative reconstructive setting.

DVT AND PE

DVT and PE are extremely morbid and potentially life-threatening complications resulting from foot and ankle reconstruction. Immobilization in the postoperative period is a predisposing factor for the development of venous thromboembolism (VTE).[30] Initiating thromboprophylaxis in patients at moderate to high VTE risk has developed into an important safety initiative along with a growing interest in identifying patients at low-risk who do not need thromboprophylaxis. These individuals may be unnecessarily subjected to the risks, costs, and inconvenience associated with such treatments.[31]

Foot and ankle reconstructive procedures do carry the potential for vascular injury, and the reconstructive surgeon must be cognizant of the Virchow triad of thrombus formation comprising venous stasis, endothelial injury, and state of hypercoagulability.[30] In contrast to more proximally situated leg surgeries, these procedures do not regularly involve the proximal deep veins and calf anatomy. Even if thrombi develop within these veins, extension into the proximal venous system, in which embolization rarely forms to cause PE, is infrequent and, in many cases, not thought to be clinically significant.[32] The more proximal the procedure, the more aggressive prophylaxis for DVT formation is generally instituted. Several components of foot and ankle reconstructive surgery should alert the surgeon and patient to the risks associated with thrombosis formation. At-risk factors include, but are not limited to, sedentary postoperative period, immobilization by casting or bracing, prevalence of diabetes and obesity, and the traumatic inflammatory processes induced by initial injury or surgery. Extended periods of non–weight bearing or limited mobility and a decrease in activity level are commonly warranted in the recovery period, causing direct association with DVT formation in this population.[33]

The lower extremity deep venous system includes the deep and superficial femoral, popliteal, sural, anterior and posterior tibial, and peroneal veins and the plantar arch. Perforating veins connect the deep and superficial network to promote flow into the deep veins during relaxation of the posterior leg muscles. Occlusion of this deep venous system by thrombosis or reflux through incompetent valves may subsequently lead to venous hypertension, and most proximal thrombi are thought to originate in the calf venous structures.[34] When thrombi involve the femoral or iliac veins, there is a higher risk of embolization, and when embolizing, the clot passes from the ileofemoral circulation through the inferior cava to the right side of the heart, where it can be pumped into the pulmonary arteries.[35] If the obstruction is large, the right ventricle cannot generate enough pressure to maintain perfusion through the pulmonary system, leading to lung segments that are ventilated but not perfused. This phenomenon may then propagate pleural effusions, pulmonary infarcts, or the inability to sufficiently oxygenate pulmonary venous return to the left side of the heart. If clots occlude enough pulmonary arterial flow, the right side of the heart may fail, thus leading to circulatory collapse and hypoxia, resulting in death.[36]

For a thrombus to congregate, venous stasis must transpire, which is a loss of proper venous function that would normally carry blood back toward the heart. This disruption is caused by injury to the veins, traumatically induced, secondary to systemic illness, or caused by a combination of multiple risk factors. In patients requiring extended periods of postoperative immobility, venous stasis occurs by 2 common phenomena. An acute deficiency of sufficient plantar flexion, leading to a decrease of calf muscle pumping for venous outflow augmentation, causes pooling of blood. Secondly, the inevitable dependent positioning of the lower extremity during periods of assisted ambulation and sitting leads to decreased venous return and blood pooling as well. In turn, these mechanisms increase venous hypertension and expression of leukocyte adhesion on the vessel endothelium, on which the circulating white blood cells and platelets may then become entangled, promoting thrombus formation.[34] During the intraoperative phase, injury to the venous endothelium may directly or indirectly occur. This action leads to the direct contact of the subendothelial collagen, further encouraging platelet and fibrin adherence and hypercoagulability. Venous stasis is elevated, and the development and extension of a thrombus may then ensue.[34] Moreover, congenital hypercoagulable conditions and other thombophilias may exist, requiring pertinent discussion before surgery.

DVT in the lower extremity presents with a deep aching pain and tightness in the calf or, possibly, thigh. If pain is experienced on active ankle dorsiflexion or resistance, it is known as Homans sign but is nonspecific and clinically unreliable.[37] Pratt sign may also be an indication for DVT, manifesting as pain or tenderness produced when squeezing the calf muscle, especially if edema and increased skin temperature is also present.[38] Systemic findings may include elevated temperature, chills, and malaise. PE symptoms can vary greatly, depending on how much of the lung is involved, the size of the clot, and the presence or absence of underlying lung disease or heart disease.[36,39] Common signs and symptoms include shortness of breath, chest pain, and cough. Definitive diagnostic testing for DVT consists of both noninvasive and invasive techniques, examples of which include the venous duplex examination and D-dimer test.[35] Testing for PE may further require computed tomography, lung ventilation or perfusion scan, or pulmonary angiography.[35] On diagnosis of DVT, various pharmacologic agents are available for treatment, some of which are adjusted-dose and low-dose unfractionated heparin, warfarin, low-molecular-weight heparin, enteric-coated aspirin, and thrombolytics.[40] Oxygen and blood pressure elevators may also be implemented.

Risk stratification is instrumental within any perioperative timeline when planning reconstructive surgery. Various factors contributing to thrombus predisposition may be acquired or may form from preexisting conditions that solely or together place the patient at risk for a thrombophilic event. Various risk factors associated with

VTE formation have been well documented, leading to the delineation of distinct risk levels.[33] Patients may be categorized as low-, moderate-, and high-risk. The surgeon must be aware of the standard circumstances commonly associated with DVT formation, such as obesity, smoking, birth control or hormone replacement therapy, varicosities, a history of DVT, hypercoagulable disorder, or active malignancy, which place the patient in the higher-risk stratum.[33,36] The foundation of risk assessment is to provide a means for initial determination for a prophylactic treatment plan; however, during the postoperative course, risk assessment must be revisited and configured for an uneventful recovery.

Felcher and colleagues[33] performed a 5-year retrospective analysis on more than 7000 patients undergoing podiatric surgery and found a DVT rate of 3 per 1000 patients and an overall rate of symptomatic PE of 0.12%. They reasserted that VTE prophylaxis continues to not be indicated for routine foot and ankle surgical procedures in patients without any additional risk factors; however, in those with a history of VTE, the risk increases to 4.6%, warranting perioperative prophylaxis.[33] They also concluded that 2 or more risk factors carried an overall VTE rate of 1.13%, which is still too low to recommend routine prophylaxis, whereas if one of those risk factors is prior VTE or the 2 risk factors are obesity and use of oral contraceptive pills, then the risk increases to roughly 5%, and VTE prophylaxis is recommended.[33] The investigators mention the limitations of the study, and they conclude that prophylactic guidelines will continue to be based on clinical judgment, observational data, and expert consensus until a prospective study is performed.

Tourniquets are commonly used in foot and ankle surgery to optimize surgical field visualization, thereby limiting operative duration and improving technical precision.[41] However, adverse events have been documented, ranging from mild skin irritation to nerve damage and paralysis, with potential for increased rates of DVT and PE.[42] Exsanguination of the limb portion is typically accomplished by elevation and/or by compression from distal to proximal up to the tourniquet site, just before tourniquet inflation, and most surgeons use an Esmarch bandage to perform the exsanguination.[41] The minimum tourniquet pressure required to safely maintain a bloodless field through limb occlusion pressure should be used in addition to a safety margin to prevent bleed-through and venous congestion. Accordingly, lower pressures reduce the risk of complications but are not as effective in maintaining hemostasis.[41]

Limb occlusion pressure is defined as the minimum tourniquet cuff pressure required to occlude arterial flow and, therefore, is measured by gradually increasing cuff pressure and noting the pressure at which distal arterial flow stops. By using the tourniquet at a lower pressure, macroscopic blood flow may be occluded but not the microcirculation, which could be beneficial for tissues to minimize capillary blockage. The most commonly used ankle-cuff pressure of 250 mm Hg and thigh-cuff pressure of 350 mm Hg are roughly based on limb occlusion pressure plus a safety margin of 40 to 60 mm Hg as reported.[41] The maximum safe periods of continuous tourniquet ischemia are most commonly considered to be 90 to 120 minutes.[41] In addition, padding support is first applied across the respective limb for additional comfort and cushioning before cuff inflation. When contemplating the use of a tourniquet, each patient and the respective procedure should be critiqued for maximum safety and efficiency.

POSTOPERATIVE INFECTION

The attentiveness in managing operative wounds for infection prophylaxis begins preoperatively. The objective is to preclude infection and other wound complications by maximizing the patient's medical stability, establishing a clean preoperative region and a sterile surgical field, using surgical techniques that minimize injury to tissues, and promptly detecting potential external causes in the postoperative setting. Infection is defined as the pathologic presence of bacteria in a wound in which the bacteria cause damage to the tissues as opposed to being harmless.[43] Infection is a clinical condition, and its diagnosis is made on clinical grounds with assistance by appropriate laboratory evaluation, when applicable. In the operative setting, factors that may influence wound contamination include insufficient antiseptic agents, inadequate sterilization of instruments or equipment, lack of proper surgical draping, increased number of operating room personnel, extended duration of surgery and/or tourniquet use, and traumatic surgical techniques.

A postoperative wound infection tends to occur within 30 days after surgery and is the most common complication in surgical patients, resulting in an average increase in hospitalization of 4 days.[44] Moreover, foot and ankle surgery may carry a higher risk of infection because the bacterial load within the operative field cannot be fully reduced. The rate of surgical site infection or deep wound infection for clean orthopedic surgical procedures is relatively low and has been reported to range from 0.008% to 17.13%.[44–46] The potential effect of a postoperative infection may be destructive, causing a delayed healing time, need for further surgery, possible loss of anatomic function or limb, permanent nerve damage and/or pain, and potential organ damage or death. Various host factors may increase the risk of surgical wound infection, such as trauma, dehydration, shock, anemia, malnutrition, and systemic conditions affecting immune compromise. Many systemic illnesses may cause an impedance of leukocytic phagocytosis, thereby lowering the body's threshold to withstand infection. The inoculum of bacteria required to cause a soft tissue infection has been estimated to be 10^5 organisms per gram.[47] In the presence of infection, cellulitis is commonly diagnosed by 1 of 5 cardinal signs including redness, swelling, pain, heat, and loss of function. When foreign invading bacteria exist, blood capillaries dilate, resulting in increased flow, which leads to the extravasation of phagocytes and fluid. Phagocyte migration is mediated by chemotactic factors, resulting in edema and, thus, stretching of nerve fibers and inevitable pain sensation.[47]

Postoperative infections are mostly associated with an inflammatory response, but it is imperative that the inflammation is attributed to an infection rather than the normal physiologic response of inflammation. Intense peri-incisional erythema, edema, heat, and pain at the surgical site should heighten the suspicion for infection. Prophylactic antibiotics may reduce infection rates in selected cases, and generally, there are certain procedural criteria recognized for improvement in infection rates when prophylaxis is implemented. These criteria include surgeries involving hardware or additional orthobiologic implementation, procedures of long duration, procedures involving extensive dissection, potential dead space formation, trauma, and patients with valvular heart disease or various other systemic illnesses.[48] The use of preoperative antibiotics for postoperative wound infection prophylaxis is a controversial issue; significant decrease in infection rates has not been shown in clean general surgical cases and nonimplant wounds.[49]

Gram-positive cocci are the most common pathogens in surgical wound infections, and the continual increase seen in multidrug resistance can create a formidable challenge for the surgeon.[46] Controlling the proliferation of drug-resistant pathogens by limiting the use of prophylactic antibiotics through accurate patient selection should be done; however, prophylactic antibiotics are often used because of their nondeleterious effects. Zgonis and colleagues[49] retrospectively reviewed 555 patients who underwent elective foot and ankle surgery, of which 306 patients received a preoperative antibiotic and 249 did not. Postoperative wound infection developed in 1.6% and 1.4% of patients who received and did not receive antibiotics, respectively.[49] Patients receiving a preoperative antibiotic had a greater tendency to develop an infection compared with patients without preoperative antibiotics. Furthermore, preoperative antibiotic use, medical history, use of internal fixation, tourniquet use, age, gender, surgical time, and surgical procedure category were not predictive of postoperative wound infections. The most common pathogens isolated were coagulase-negative and coagulase-positive staphylococci.[49]

The due diligence in implementing antimicrobial chemoprophylaxis in clean orthopedic surgery has not yet been agreed on, yet many surgeons administer preoperative antibiotics in complicated and prolonged cases. Diabetes mellitus is of particular interest when contemplating the risk assessment for postoperative infections. The number of people affected is steadily increasing, with approximately 7.6% of the US population, or 23.6 million people, being diagnosed.[50] Furthermore, people older than 65 years constitute 38% of this subpopulation.[50] As a result, foot and ankle surgeons are more readily exposed to these patients because of the high prevalence of foot and ankle infections experienced by this subset. Wukich and colleagues[51] conducted a recent study hypothesizing that the infection rate in the diabetic population would be higher than that in patients without diabetes, in addition to expecting to see a higher risk for postoperative infection in persons with a more advanced disease state. The overall infection rate was 4.8% in a series of 1000 patients, with 2.8% in the control group and 13.2% in the diabetic study group. Patients with a more advanced disease state had a 10-fold greater risk of infection compared with nondiabetic patients and a 6-fold greater risk compared with patients with uncomplicated diabetes.[51] The investigators demonstrated that a history of diabetes mellitus significantly increases the risk for severe infection, requiring hospitalization and/or further surgical intervention.

If an infection presents in the postoperative period, empiric antibiotics should be promptly initiated based on the clinical state, experience in determining the likely pathogen, and Gram stain results, if deemed reliable. Radiograph evaluation should be done depending on the time elapsed for the detection of osseous changes or soft tissue emphysema. Imaging studies may be warranted, with bone scans not providing much guidance because of low specificity; however, magnetic resonance imaging may offer greater exactness and insight for infection evaluation. The treating physician should also evaluate any bacteria and antibiotic sensitivity reports from the institution employed, with special regard to resistant strain identification. The infection may subsequently warrant additional decompression, drainage, or debridement for additional recovery. Cognizance of all potential sources of infection and an expedited identification and treatment are paramount in the perioperative setting.

REHABILITATION OBSTACLES

When supervising reconstructive surgeries in the postoperative phase, acknowledgment must be made to the degree of surgery, severity, healing time, and level of return to activity. Furthermore, it is imperative to scrutinize the improved foot type created if applicable, altered biomechanics, footwear worn during expected activity, and need for external supports, such as bracing or taping. Rehabilitation is aimed at enabling patients to reach and maintain their optimal physical, sensory, intellectual, psychological, and social functional levels. In patients who may have been debilitated for an extended duration, independence and self-determination are central to the restoration of function and return to activities of daily living.

Most patients undergoing foot and ankle reconstructive surgery require a period of immobilization and limited activity. This restriction may cause major inconveniences to the patients because they are incapacitated and unable to care for themselves in most instances. A period of non–weight bearing normally includes application of a short-leg posterior splint or cast, whereas more complicated reconstructive procedures may require a multiplane circular external fixator. The course of immobilization routinely extends from 6 to 8 weeks, with a longer duration for more comprehensive reconstruction. A course of partial or limited weight bearing may then follow, and the patient is allowed to wear a walking boot or brace before finally transitioning to a supportive shoe, with continued ambulatory restrictions. The healing time layout may be extensive but integral for normalization of the extremity for reestablishment of distal perfusion, venous pump activation, increase of capillary inflow, and restoration of muscle, tendon, and ligament strength. The surgeon must continue to be perceptive of potential complications during this period that may notably impair the recovery process. Prominent drawbacks include, and are not limited to, delayed union, malunion, and nonunion of osseous reconstruction, as well as skin incision dehiscence. These phenomena subsequently alter the decision-making process for further treatment in the postoperative setting.

For extensive procedures, usually those involving rearfoot deformity correction or limb salvage attempts, patients are admitted to the hospital for approximately 3 to 7 days to properly control postoperative edema and pain in the acute setting. IV antibiotics are routinely extended through this period as well, with orders for strict bed rest and extremity elevation. In addition, the postoperative hospital stay allows for close monitoring of any comorbidities, ensuring that the patient is medically stable and able to rehabilitate before discharge, ideally becoming capable for bed to chair transfer and minimal, short-duration assisted ambulation with crutches or walker. Social workers and case management teams are called on for assistance in placement to skilled-nursing facilities to further closely monitored care. The extent of reconstruction involved and the ultimate patient confinement, presence of comorbidities, and evaluation of overall body strength are mediating variables that are meticulously evaluated. A patient's significant other, family member, or friend is often requested to provide support pertaining to assistance in the patient's home, facilitating transportation, or simply being available for companionship.

The physical therapy team is instrumental in aiding the rehabilitation of the patients. Physical therapy is a well-established modality for the restoration of function after disorders of the musculoskeletal system, and nearly all foot and ankle reconstructive surgeries may benefit from rehabilitation programs that include therapeutic exercise. Restoring joint range of motion when applicable, muscle strength, and neuromuscular coordination need to be emphasized, as should normal gait mechanics. A graduated return to physical activity that includes function-specific movement is recommended, with the primary goal being a safe return to motion while minimizing the risk of recurrent pathologic condition or pain.

SUMMARY

All surgical procedures carry potential complications. Perioperative management is paramount in anticipating unfavorable experiences for both the patient and the surgeon. Meticulous postoperative care is essential and should be a priority of the entire treatment team and associated professionals to prevent such complications.

REFERENCES

1. Thompson JS, Baxter BT, Allison JG, et al. Temporal patterns of postoperative complications. Arch Surg 2003;138:596–602.

2. Butterworth P, Gilheany MF, Tinley P. Postoperative infection rates in foot and ankle surgery: a clinical audit of Australian podiatric surgeons, January to December 2007. Aust Health Rev 2010;34:180–5.

3. Dolin SJ, Cashman JN. Tolerability of acute postoperative pain management: nausea, vomiting, sedation, pruritus, and urinary retention. Evidence from published data. Br J Anaesth 2005;95:584–91.

4. Scholz J, Woolf CJ. Can we conquer pain? Nat Neurosci 2002;5(Suppl): 1062–7.

5. Souzdalnitski D, Halaszynski TM, Faclier G. Regional anesthesia and co-existing chronic pain. Curr Opin Anaesthesiol 2010;23:662–70.

6. Carr DB, Goudas LC. Acute pain. Lancet 1999;353:2051–8.

7. Pflug AE, Bonica JJ. Physiopathology and control of postoperative pain. Arch Surg 1977;112:773–81.

8. Gold BS, Kitz DS, Lecky JH, et al. Unanticipated admission to the hospital following ambulatory surgery. JAMA 1989;262:3008–10.

9. Shirakami G, Teratani Y, Namba T, et al. Delayed discharge and acceptability of ambulatory surgery in adult outpatients receiving general anesthesia. J Anesth 2005;19:93–101.

10. White PF, Kehlet H. Postoperative pain management and patient outcome: time to return to work! Anesth Analg 2007;104:487–9.

11. Woolf CJ, Salter MW. Neuronal plasticity: increasing the gain in pain. Science 2000;288:1765–9.

12. Reilley TE, Gerhardt MA. Anesthesia for foot and ankle surgery. Clin Podiatr Med Surg 2002;19:125–47.

13. Chelly JE, Greger J, Casati A, et al. Continuous lateral sciatic blocks for acute postoperative pain management after major ankle and foot surgery. Foot Ankle Int 2002;23:749–52.

14. Hunt KJ, Higgins TF, Carlston CV, et al. Continuous peripheral nerve blockade as postoperative analgesia for open treatment of calcaneal fractures. J Orthop Trauma 2010;24:148–55.

15. Mabee J, Orlinsky M. Bier block exsanguination: a volumetric comparison and venous pressure study. Acad Emerg Med 2000;7:105–13.

16. Fischer SP. Development and effectiveness of an anesthesia preoperative evaluation clinic in a teaching hospital. Anesthesiology 1996;85:196–206.

17. Jenkins K, Baker AB. Consent and anaesthetic risk. Anaesthesia 2003;58: 962–84.

18. Varitimidis SE, Venouziou AI, Dailiana ZH, et al. Triple nerve block at the knee for foot and ankle surgery performed by the surgeon: difficulties and efficiency. Foot Ankle Int 2009;30:854–9.

19. Ganzberg S, Kramer KJ. The use of local anesthetic agents in medicine. Dent Clin North Am 2010;54:601–10.

20. Clough TM, Sandher D, Bale RS, et al. The use of a local anesthetic foot block in patients undergoing outpatient bony forefoot surgery: a prospective randomized controlled trial. J Foot Ankle Surg 2003;42:24–9.

21. Kapitanyan R, Su M. Toxicity, local anesthetics. Available at: http://emedicine. medscape.com/article/819628-overview. Accessed August 28, 2010.

22. Chowdhry S, Seidenstricker L, Cooney DS, et al. Do not use epinephrine in digital blocks: myth or truth? Part II, a retrospective review of 1,111 cases. Plast Reconstr Surg 2010. [Epub ahead of print].

23. Sarrafian SK, Ibrahim IN, Breihan JH. Ankle-foot peripheral nerve block for mid and forefoot surgery. Foot Ankle 1983;4:86–90.

24. Ribotsky BM, Berkowitz KD, Montague JR. Local anesthetics. Is there an advantage to mixing solutions? J Am Podiatr Med Assoc 1996;86:487–91.
25. Langford RM. Pain management today—what have we learned? Clin Rheumatol 2006;25(Suppl 1):S2–8.
26. Bassols A, Bosch F, Baños JE. How does the general population treat their pain? A survey in Catalonia, Spain. J Pain Symptom Manage 2002;23:318–28.
27. Phero JC, Becker DE, Dionne RA. Contemporary trends in acute pain management. Curr Opin Otolaryngol Head Neck Surg 2004;12:209–16.
28. Grass JA. Patient-controlled analgesia. Anesth Analg 2005;101:S44–61.
29. Schein JR, Hicks RW, Nelson WW, et al. Patient-controlled analgesia-related medication errors in the postoperative period: causes and prevention. Drug Saf 2009;32:549–59.
30. Geerts WH, Bergqvist D, Pineo GF, et al. Prevention of venous thromboembolism: American College of Chest Physicians Evidence-Based Clinical Practice Guidelines (8th edition). Chest 2008;133(Suppl 6):381S–453S.
31. Virchow R. [Neuer fall von tod licher embolic der lungenarterian]. Arch Pathol Anat 1856;10:225–8 [in German].
32. Kearon C. Natural history of venous thromboembolism. Circulation 2003;107:I22–30.
33. Felcher AH, Mularski RA, Mosen DM, et al. Incidence and risk factors for venous thromboembolic disease in podiatric surgery. Chest 2009;135:917–22.
34. Gschwandtner ME, Ehringer H. Microcirculation in chronic venous insufficiency. Vasc Med 2001;6:169–79.
35. Slaybaugh RS, Beasley BD, Massa EG. Deep venous thrombosis risk assessment, incidence, and prophylaxis in foot and ankle surgery. Clin Podiatr Med Surg 2003;20:269–89.
36. Mantilla CB, Horlocker TT, Schroeder DR, et al. Frequency of myocardial infarction, pulmonary embolism, deep venous thrombosis, and death following primary hip or knee arthroplasty. Anesthesiology 2002;96:1140–6.
37. Ng KC. Deep vein thrombosis: a study in clinical diagnosis. Singapore Med J 1994;35:286–9.
38. Julsrud ME. A review of the birth control pill and its relationship to thrombophlebitis. J Am Podiatr Med Assoc 1979;69:376–82.
39. Parvizi J, Jacovides CL, Bican O, et al. Is deep vein thrombosis a good proxy for pulmonary embolus? J Arthroplasty 2010;25(Suppl 6):138–44.
40. Osinbowale O, Ali L, Chi YW. Venous thromboembolism: a clinical review. Postgrad Med 2010;122:54–65.
41. Kalla TP, Younger A, McEwen JA, et al. Survey of tourniquet use in podiatric surgery. J Foot Ankle Surg 2003;42:68–76.
42. Smith TO, Hing CB. The efficacy of the tourniquet in foot and ankle surgery? A systematic review and meta-analysis. Foot Ankle Surg 2010;16:3–8.
43. Wilson AP, Livesey SA, Treasure T, et al. Factors predisposing to wound infection in cardiac surgery. A prospective study of 517 patients. Eur J Cardiothorac Surg 1987;1:158–64.
44. Neumayer L, Hosokawa P, Itani K, et al. Multivariable predictors of postoperative surgical site infection after general and vascular surgery: results from the Patient Safety in Surgery Study. J Am Coll Surg 2007;204:1178–87.
45. Trampuz A, Zimmerli W. Antimicrobial agents in orthopaedic surgery: prophylaxis and treatment. Drugs 2006;66:1089–105.
46. Cantlon CA, Stemper ME, Schwan WR, et al. Significant pathogens isolated from surgical site infections at a community hospital in the Midwest. Am J Infect Control 2006;34:526–9.

47. Siddiqui AR, Bernstein JM. Chronic wound infection: facts and controversies. Clin Dermatol 2010;28:519–26.
48. Kaiser AB. Postoperative infectious and antimicrobial prophylaxis. In: Mandell GL, Douglas RG, Bennett JE, editors. Principles and practice of infectious disease. 3rd edition. New York: Churchill Livingstone; 1990. p. 2245–57.
49. Zgonis T, Jolly GP, Garbalosa JC. The efficacy of prophylactic intravenous antibiotics in elective foot and ankle surgery. J Foot Ankle Surg 2004;43:97–103.
50. Centers for Disease Control and Prevention. National diabetes fact sheet: general information and national estimates on diabetes in the United States, 2007. Atlanta (GA): US Department of Health and Human Services, Centers for Disease Control and Prevention; 2008.
51. Wukich DK, Lowery NJ, McMillen RL, et al. Postoperative infection rates in foot and ankle surgery: a comparison of patients with and without diabetes mellitus. J Bone Joint Surg Am 2010;92:287–95.

Index

Note: Page numbers of article titles are in **boldface** type.

A

Abscesses, 27–30
Acellular products, for bone healing, 55–56
Acetaminophen, 79–80
Achilles tendon lengthening, for pediatric flatfoot, 3–4
Alloderm, 55
Allogenic orthobiologics, 52–53
Ambulatory surgery, pain control in, 76
Amputation
    for diabetic foot, 30
    for trauma, 35–38
Analgesia, patient-controlled, 80
Anesthesia
    anatomic considerations in, 78
    complications of, 76
    for elective surgery, 2
    for hallux valgus correction, 3
    for infection surgery, 31
    for pediatric flatfoot correction, 4
    for plastic surgery, 48
    for rearfoot arthrodesis, 5
    for rheumatoid arthritis, 12
    for trauma repair, 38
    general, 77
    local, 77–79
    regional, 77–79
    selection of, 77–79
Angiography, for peripheral vascular disease, 19–21
Angioplasty, for peripheral vascular disease, 22
Ankle block, 78
Ankle surgery. *See* Foot and ankle surgery.
Ankle-brachial index, for peripheral vascular disease, 18–19
Antibiotics
    after elective surgery, 6
    after peripheral vascular disease surgery, 23–24
    after rheumatoid arthritis surgery, 14
    after trauma repair, 39
    before plastic surgery, 47
    for abscess, 27
    for Charcot neuroarthropathy, 70
    for osteomyelitis, 27
    for trauma, 37

Perioperative Nursing Clinics 6 (2011) 89–99
doi:10.1016/S1556-7931(10)00106-3
periopnursing.theclinics.com
1556-7931/11/$ – see front matter © 2011 Elsevier Inc. All rights reserved.

Moving?

Make sure your subscription moves with you!

To notify us of your new address, find your **Clinics Account Number** (located on your mailing label above your name), and contact customer service at:

Email: journalscustomerservice-usa@elsevier.com

800-654-2452 (subscribers in the U.S. & Canada)
314-447-8871 (subscribers outside of the U.S. & Canada)

Fax number: 314-447-8029

Elsevier Health Sciences Division
Subscription Customer Service
3251 Riverport Lane
Maryland Heights, MO 63043

*To ensure uninterrupted delivery of your subscription, please notify us at least 4 weeks in advance of move.